# Endorsemen

*Dr. Patrick Foye is a leading international expert at evaluating and treating tailbone pain. His coccyx patients come from around the world. He publishes and lectures extensively on this topic. His book,* Tailbone Pain Relief Now!, *will certainly help those who are afflicted by tailbone pain worldwide.*

**—John R. Bach, M.D.**, Professor and Vice Chairman, Physical Medicine and Rehabilitation, Rutgers New Jersey Medical School

*If you have tailbone pain as I do, this book could save you years of pain and suffering. I highly recommend it for anyone with coccyx problems.*

**—Maria T.**, attorney, California

*This book explains everything that I needed to learn about my tailbone injury. It's easy to read and understand, even though I don't have any medical training.* **—Margaret C.**, customer service representative, New York

Tailbone Pain Relief Now! *helped me understand what is causing my coccyx pain and the best options for treating it.*

**—Christopher L.**, police officer, Florida

# Patrick M. Foye, M.D.

# Tailbone Pain Relief Now!

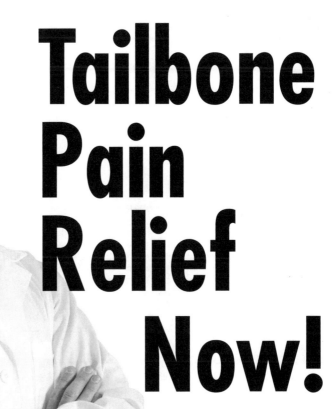

## Causes and Treatments for Your Sore or Injured Coccyx

Top Quality Publishing, LLC

Bulk copies of this book may be purchased by contacting
the publisher directly at: info@TopQualityPublishing.com

Publisher: Top Quality Publishing, LLC
Cover and interior design: Rebecca Finkel, F+P Graphic Design
Book Consultant: Judith Briles, The Book Shepherd
Editor: John Maling, Editing by John
Illustrations: Don Sidle, DonSidle.net
Cover photo: Doug Zacker, ZackerImages.com

Library of Congress Catalog Number: on file
ISBN: 978-0-9964535-0-9
ebook ISBN: 978-0-9964535-1-6

Foye, Patrick M.
*Tailbone Pain Relief Now! Causes and Treatments for Your Sore or Injured Coccyx.*
Categories for cataloging and shelving:
1. Health | Musculoskeletal  2. Pain Management
3. Tailbone pain  4. Coccyx pain  5. Back pain

10  9  8  7  6  5  4  3  2  1

# Contents

**PART ONE** Finding the Cause of Your Tailbone Pain ............7

**1** Introduction ......................................................9

**2** Symptoms of Tailbone Pain (Coccyx Pain) ................... 15

**3** Overcoming Stigma: Psychology of Tailbone Pain .......... 23

**4** Anatomy of Tailbone Pain ..................................... 29

**5** Causes of Tailbone Pain ....................................... 37

**6** Unstable Tailbone Joints: Dynamic Instability ............... 39

**7** Tailbone Fractures: The Broken Coccyx ...................... 51

**8** Dislocations of the Tailbone .................................. 59

**9** Bone Spurs of the Tailbone ................................... 65

**10** Arthritis of the Tailbone ........................................ 71

**11** Abnormal Position of the Tailbone ........................... 75

**12** Sympathetic Nervous System Pain at the Coccyx ........... 79

**13** Cancer Causing Tailbone Pain ............................... 85

**14** Bone Infection Causing Coccyx Pain ......................... 93

**15** Back and Buttock Pain ....................................... 103

**16** Medical Tests for Tailbone Pain ............................. 115

**17** Consultations with Other Medical Specialists.............. 131

**PART TWO** Treatments to Relieve Your Tailbone Pain ....... 139

**18** Treatments for Tailbone Pain: Overview.................... 141

**19** Avoid Worsening Your Tailbone Pain....................... 145

**20** Cushions for Tailbone Pain ................................. 151

**21** Medications for Tailbone Pain............................. 159

**22** Manipulation of the Coccyx ............................... 169

**23** Exercise and Tailbone Pain................................. 175

**24** Injections for Tailbone Pain................................. 181

**25** Coccygectomy: Surgical Removal of the Tailbone ........ 195


**PART THREE** Special Situations Regarding Tailbone Pain .. 201

**26** Working with Your Doctors................................. 203

**27** Pregnancy, Childbirth and Tailbone Pain.................. 215

**28** Children with Tailbone Pain ............................... 223

**29** Health Insurance for Tailbone Pain ....................... 227

**30** Legal Cases for Tailbone Injuries ......................... 239


**PART FOUR** Book Summary ................................... 243

**31** Take Home Points .......................................... 245

Come for Medical Care from Dr. Foye............................ 247

Testimonials from Dr. Foye's Patients............................ 249

About the Author .................................................. 251

Acknowledgments ................................................. 253

Bibliography/References ........................................... 255

Index ............................................................... 263

Free Bonuses for You.............................................. 269

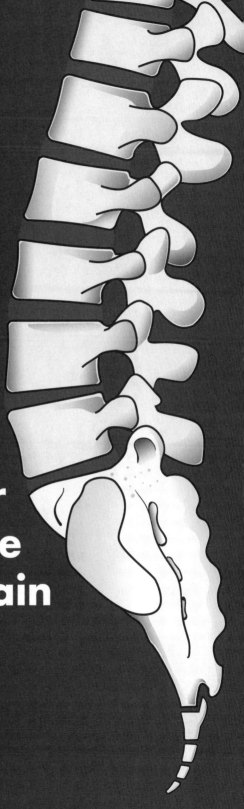

PART ONE

# Finding the Cause of Your Tailbone Pain

## In This Section

**1** Introduction.............................. 9

**2** Symptoms of Tailbone Pain
(Coccyx Pain)........................... 15

**3** Overcoming Stigma:
Psychology of Tailbone Pain.......... 23

**4** Anatomy of Tailbone Pain............. 29

**5** Causes of Tailbone Pain............... 37

**6** Unstable Tailbone Joints:
Dynamic Instability .................... 39

**7** Tailbone Fractures:
the Broken Coccyx .................... 51

**8** Dislocations of the Tailbone........... 59

**9** Bone Spurs of the Tailbone........... 65

**10** Arthritis of the Tailbone............... 71

**11** Abnormal Position of the Tailbone....75

**12** Sympathetic Nervous System
Pain at the Coccyx .................... 79

**13** Cancer Causing Tailbone Pain ....... 85

**14** Bone Infection Causing
Tailbone Pain .......................... 93

**15** Back and Buttock Pain.............. 103

**16** Medical Tests for Tailbone Pain..... 115

**17** Consults with
Other Medical Specialists .......... 131

# CHAPTER 1

# Introduction

## Who is This Book for?

If you are suffering from tailbone pain (coccyx pain), this book is for you. If you want answers for what is causing your tailbone pain, this book is for you. If you want relief from tailbone pain, this book is for you.

*Tailbone Pain Relief Now!* will help you and empower you. In this book you will discover the knowledge you

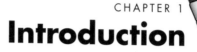

**Tailbone Pain Relief Now! is for you, the person with tailbone pain.**

need to understand your tailbone pain symptoms, diagnostic tests and treatment options. You will discover multiple pathways to relief from pain.

Since many of you may not be able to make the trip to see me in person at our Tailbone Pain Center, this book is my way of helping even those who I may never meet in person. Every week in my clinical practice I meet patients who have suffered with tailbone pain for months or years without answers and without relief. For every patient who has flown in to see me from another state or another country, there are probably hundreds and thousands more who also need the information in this book.

*Tailbone Pain Relief Now!* will help you to diplomatically approach your treating physicians with the right questions and suggestions so that your doctors can better help you, even if they are not very familiar with treating tailbone pain.

You can also find additional patient education materials on my website: **TailboneDoctor.com**. But this book allows for a thorough and well-organized presentation that you can read offline and bring right to your doctor's office. You can highlight or underline the parts that apply to you. You can make notes in the margins. You can refer back to it as often as needed if your tailbone pain continues.

I initially considered writing this book mainly for doctors, rather than for patients. I'm an academic physician (a medical school Professor) who has worked in medical education for more than 20 years. I've spent decades educating medical students, interns, resident physicians, attending physicians, peers and colleagues. I've published in peer-reviewed medical journals, given grand rounds presentations at hospitals in many states, presented at national medical conferences, and written book chapters about tailbone pain in various medical textbooks. So I have spent my career educating doctors. (For more information on my history, *see* About the Author.)

Unfortunately, my patients who come to see me from around the country and around the world tell me that the medical knowledge is simply not trickling down well enough or fast enough to their local physicians. Even the most caring and well-intentioned doctors are unable to stay up-to-date on every single medical condition affecting their patients. This is especially true for conditions that are relatively uncommon, such as tailbone pain.

So *Tailbone Pain Relief Now!* is for you, the person with tailbone pain. My goal here is to put the knowledge you need directly into your hands. With knowledge comes hope: hope for answers, hope

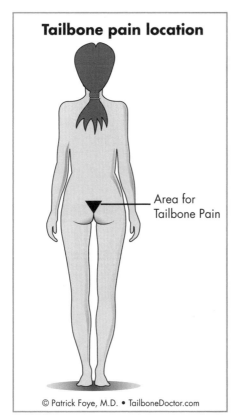

**Tailbone pain location**

Area for Tailbone Pain

© Patrick Foye, M.D. • TailboneDoctor.com

for relief, and hope for restoration of your quality of life. These hopes can become a reality. Knowledge is power. *Tailbone Pain Relief Now!* puts that power in your hands.

## Dr. Foye's Personal Share

Many patients ask me how I became interested in treating tailbone pain and whether I ever suffered from it. I have not, but the background answer is more complex than that. It involves my son's rare medical condition, which does not even involve the coccyx. But it does involve seeking medical expertise that was hard to find.

After my son was born in 2001, he was diagnosed with a rare condition that incorrectly gave a predicted life expectancy of only one to two years. My wife and I were frustrated that most physicians had never seen a patient with his condition, and even the experts had never before seen his particular form. So I have experienced your despair of having physicians who are not experienced at treating the condition that you or your family need help with.

My son is now a happy, fun and bright teenager. But he still faces ongoing medical challenges due to a condition that few doctors have ever seen before. We learned the importance of finding the right specialist and the right information.

Meanwhile, I had already published medical papers on various musculoskeletal and pain topics including tailbone pain. Patients with tailbone pain who found me and came for treatment often described prior frustrations with inexperienced doctors. I recognized that I could make the positive difference for tailbone patients, just as my wife and I sought doctors with expertise to make a positive difference for our son's rare condition.

So I created the Tailbone Pain Center. Treating patients with tailbone pain has absolutely turned out to be the most personally gratifying part of my career as a physician. My patients have taught me more than all of the countless medical journals and books I have read. Now I am writing this book to share what I have learned, to help those with tailbone pain.

I have published more than 30 medical articles, chapters, and abstracts specifically on the topic of tailbone pain in previous medical journals and books for physicians. Here, in *Tailbone Pain Relief Now!*, I summarize almost two decades of my medical publications (and those of others). I convert medical jargon written for physicians into language and explanations geared specifically for patients. My goal is that this book will help as many people as possible.

## What Format Will this Book Follow?

*Tailbone Pain Relief Now!* will start by helping you discover what you need to know about tailbone pain symptoms, terminology, and basic anatomy. Next, this book will reveal the diagnostic tests that are helpful in evaluating tailbone pain. Then we will explore many available treatment options that can provide relief. Lastly, we will cover special situations, such as tailbone pain during pregnancy or during childhood.

Most chapters start with a story of a person who I have treated for tailbone pain. Of course, within this book patient names and other details have been changed to protect patient confidentiality. Many of their stories may sound familiar to you and may be similar to what you have been experiencing with your own tailbone pain.

Many chapters include links to my website that provide you with additional, bonus content available as my free online gifts for readers. These include checklists and other useful resources that will help you and your doctors to navigate your way through the best available tests and treatments for tailbone pain.

The bibliography at the end of the book will list the main source materials from the published medical literature.

## Limits and Disclaimers

*Tailbone Pain Relief Now!* is for educational or informational purposes only. This book is not to be considered as specific medical advice or treatment for any one specific person. There is no "doctor-patient relationship" between myself and readers (except for those who actually come to see me in person, in which case my in-person advice trumps the general information presented in this book).

My purpose is to empower patients with thorough and up-to-date knowledge about tests and treatments for tailbone pain. But this book, in itself, is not a substitute for in-person medical care from a physician. No book or website can replace the benefits of in-person medical care from a medical doctor who has knowledge and experience evaluating and treating tailbone pain.

None of the tests or treatments in this book are "guaranteed" to provide the most accurate diagnosis or provide complete and sustained relief of pain. But after more than 20 years as a physician with literally thousands of patient visits related to tailbone pain, I believe this book will provide the best available book-form resource for patients with coccyx pain.

While this book is thorough, it cannot include every detail I've learned from thousands of patient visits for tailbone pain. So, the book will focus on delivering the knowledge likely to be most helpful for the vast majority of tailbone pain patients.

Also, new medical research continually emerges. But this book gives you a current snapshot at the time of publication. After reading this book, you will probably be more knowledgeable and up-to-date on the topic of tailbone pain than your local physicians.

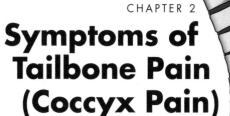

# CHAPTER 2

# Symptoms of Tailbone Pain (Coccyx Pain)

## Jennifer's Story

Jennifer was thrilled that her recent promotion had her advancing smoothly up the corporate ladder. But she started having pain in the middle of her lower buttocks area while sitting, especially if she sat leaning slightly backward. Her pain was worse while she went from sitting to standing. She never had pain in this area before and was unsure what could be causing it. Most of her day was spent sitting, all the while suffering in pain. The pain caused difficulties with sitting during her commute, during meetings at work, and while trying to get work done sitting at her computer. The pain caused her to lose focus at work. She spent a lot of time and mental energy trying to figure out what chairs were the least painful to sit on. She often sat leaning toward one side or the other, or sat leaning forward, to minimize the pain. Her local doctor mislabeled her as having "low back pain," but Jennifer knew her symptoms were lower down. After months of suffering she eventually discovered that she had tailbone pain (coccyx pain) and came to our Tailbone Pain Center for evaluation and successful treatment. Her symptoms were typical for tailbone pain.

## Terms: Tailbone Pain, Coccyx Pain, Coccydynia, Coccygodynia

The terms tailbone pain, coccyx pain, coccydynia, and coccygodynia all mean the same thing. All of these terms simply refer to pain at the tailbone (coccyx). The tailbone, or coccyx, is the lowest group of bones within the human spine. Physicians more commonly use the term coccyx, while patients often use the term tailbone, but both are talking about the same thing.

Meanwhile, medical words ending with "-dynia" are referring to pain. So, the terms coccydynia (coccy-dynia) and coccygodynia (coccygo-dynia) simply mean coccyx pain.

Note that a term or phrase like coccyx pain or coccydynia is still just describing a symptom (what the patient is feeling). None of these terms actually explain what is causing this pain. The causes of tailbone pain will be addressed in later chapters within this book, beginning with Chapter 5, *Causes of Tailbone Pain*.

## What Makes Tailbone Pain Worse?

Sitting typically makes tailbone pain worse. When you sit, the weight from the upper half of your body presses down through your pelvis. Three bony areas in the lower pelvis form a "tripod" to bear this body weight. These three bones are the ischial bones (one at the bottom of each buttock, right and left) and, in the midline, the tailbone. The ischial bones are sometimes called the "sit bones" (or sitting bones), but the tailbone should also be considered a sit bone.

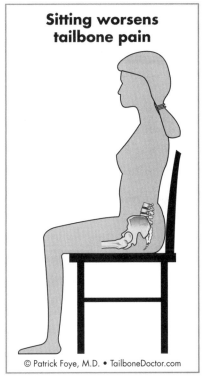

**Sitting worsens tailbone pain**

© Patrick Foye, M.D. • TailboneDoctor.com

Although tailbone pain can be worsened by activities other than sitting, pain with sitting is the most common feature.

Tailbone pain is also usually worsened by pressing directly on the tailbone, which your physician can do during the physical exam, or you can even do it by yourself in seeking to confirm the source of your pain.

## Sitting Leaning Backward

Leaning partway backward (slightly reclining) while sitting generally makes tailbone pain even worse than sitting straight up. The reason is that when we sit leaning backward we put more of our body weight onto the back part of the pelvis (where the tailbone is) rather than the front part of the pelvis.

## Sitting Leaning Forward

As noted above, when sitting leaning

**Sitting typically makes tailbone pain worse.**

partway backward more of your body weight is put upon your tailbone. The opposite is also true. If while sitting you flex forward at the hips and waist, more of your body weight shifts to the front part of the pelvis and away from the tailbone at the back area of the pelvis. So while sitting, tailbone pain is often relieved by leaning forward.

Unfortunately, leaning forward while sitting can eventually cause musculoskeletal pain in other body regions. These additional problems will be discussed in detail in Chapter 15: *Back and Buttock Pain.*

## Sitting Leaning Toward One Side (Right or Left)

When you sit leaning to one side (either to the right or to the left), the pressure of your body weight shifts away from your tailbone, which is at the midline. So, patients with tailbone pain will often sit either leaning forward (as discussed above) or leaning toward the right or left side.

Unfortunately, this usually provides only partial relief and, over time, sitting in such an abnormal position (leaning toward one side or the other) causes stresses that can result in musculoskeletal pain in other body regions (such as the ischial bursa and the piriformis muscle, which will be discussed in Chapter 15).

## Increased Pain When Going from Sitting to Standing

Some people with tailbone pain experience a sudden, dramatic, temporary worsening of their pain during the few seconds that it takes to go from sitting to standing. There are many reasons for this.

First, many people with tailbone pain have unstable joints within the tailbone. This is called dynamic instability of the coccyx. "Instability" means that the joints are unstable (too loose, too lax) between the individual bones of the coccyx. This is a very common cause of tailbone pain, but unfortunately many physicians are unaware of this phenomenon. When you are sitting, the additional body weight pressing down upon your tailbone causes any unstable joints to undergo excessive movement. Your joints may flex too much, or extend too much, or they may go into a partially or completely dislocated position. This is the nature of dynamic instability, which will be discussed in detail in Chapter 6: *Unstable Tailbone Joints: Dynamic Instability.*

The unstable coccygeal joints are often even more painful when the patient stands up (because then the coccygeal bones abruptly, suddenly shift back into a more normal alignment). This is similar to a shoulder dislocation, which is temporarily even more painful while the shoulder is being relocated back into its normal position.

Worsening coccyx pain when going from sitting to standing may also be caused by things other than unstable joints of the tailbone. The transition from sitting to standing may involve rocking your body weight as you get up, temporarily causing increased pressure on your tailbone. Also while rising, various muscles begin to activate (contract) including some muscles that attach to the tailbone and this puts additional stress or pull upon the tailbone.

## Where Is Your Tailbone?

Many people have worse body awareness for anatomic structures within their pelvis than they do for other body regions. For example, if I asked you to point to (or describe the location of) your biceps muscle, or the farthest joint (knuckle) on your pinky finger, you would have no difficulty doing so. But if I asked you to point to or describe the location of your coccygeus muscle or the lowest joint on your coccyx, you probably would have substantial difficulty doing so. This can create challenges for patients with tailbone pain, since they may not be sure whether the pain is really coming from the tailbone or not.

The tailbone is the lowest region of the human spine. It is located in the midline below the sacrum and above the anus. If you use your finger to press externally below your sacrum and above your anus, at the midline "crack" between the right and left buttock muscles, you will probably be able to feel a small bony hardness there. This is the tailbone. If this is the location of your pain, then most likely you have coccydynia (tailbone pain). You may be able to reproduce your pain by pressing specifically on this area.

Ideally, your physician should be able to help you with making this determination. You can point specifically to the area of pain, or even mark the skin there with a marker in advance of that physician visit, and ask the doctor to confirm whether this is the tailbone that is painful. Admittedly, many physicians are not knowledgeable or experienced in evaluating tailbone pain, but hopefully this guided approach can help you move your assessment in the right direction.

## Tailbone Pain Traveling to Other Body Regions

Similar to other musculoskeletal and neurologic pains, tailbone pain can sometimes travel (or "refer" or "radiate") to other nearby body regions. But usually tailbone pain stays focal specifically at the tailbone itself.

So, while pain in the adjacent nearby musculoskeletal areas *might* be referred from the tailbone, it is very possible that the pain in those other areas might *not* be coming from the tailbone pain at all. A thorough medical evaluation is necessary to assess for the source of pain in each different location.

For example, pain in the anal or rectal area, including pain with bowel movements (while passing stool) certainly could be due to a tailbone problem, but is more likely to be coming from an anal or rectal problem. Consultation with a gastroenterologist may be needed.

Pain in the genital region at the front of the pelvis (including the vaginal region in women and the scrotum and penis in men) warrants further evaluation beyond just the tailbone. Consultation with an obstetrician/gynecologist or a urologist may be worthwhile in such cases.

Similarly, in cases where a substantial amount of the pain is at the right or left buttock (gluteal region), or down either leg, it is medically necessary to consider sources of pain other than just the tailbone.

In summary, tailbone pain usually stays focal, localized at the tailbone, and when it does travel, it usually only does so to the limited area close to the tailbone. The further away from the tailbone pain you feel symptoms, the more likely it is that those symptoms are being caused by something *other* than tailbone pain. Pain at those other sites may be separate from, and in addition to, the pain at your tailbone. These other painful sites are discussed in greater depth in Chapter 15: *Back and Buttock Pain.*

**Free Bonus for You**

For your free copy of the Tailbone Pain Symptom Checklist, go to: **TailboneDoctor.com/forms**

# CHAPTER 3

# Overcoming Stigma: Psychology of Tailbone Pain

## Lisa's Story

Lisa felt awkward and embarrassed about the pain she was having between her buttocks, just above her anus. When she told her physician that she thought she had coccyx pain he chuckled out loud. Lisa wondered why he would laugh about her pain and suffering. She felt hurt by his insensitive attitude but she kept her emotions inside. Without doing any physical examination, her doctor dismissively told her she was probably just experiencing anxiety and stress. He offhandedly suggested that the pain was just "in her head" and recommended relaxing meditation and medications to treat anxiety, neither of which helped her pain.

Lisa began to feel frustrated. Her life started to revolve around how she could avoid worsening her pain. The pain drained her energy. She became easily irritated with her husband, children, friends, and coworkers. She became withdrawn. She sometimes cried, alone. Eventually, she came to our Tailbone Pain Center, where we confirmed that her pain was not just "in her head," it was in her tailbone. Tailbone x-rays done while she was sitting showed clear and objective evidence of an unstable joint at her tailbone (see Chapter 6: *Unstable Tailbone Joints: Dynamic Instability*). Learning what was causing her condition (and that it was treatable) gave her dramatic emotional relief.

Unfortunately, there is substantial stigma against patients with tailbone pain and other pelvic pain syndromes.

Societal norms consider the pelvic region to be an area for modesty and discretion. Some older or stricter societal norms unfortunately go further and consider medical conditions in the pelvic region to be somehow dirty or taboo topics, not to be discussed.

Even the word "pudendal" comes from a Latin word meaning "parts to be ashamed of." In medicine, "pudendal" is the name of the nerve that innervates much of the pelvis, especially the genital region. It implies that the pelvic region is a site for not just modesty, but rather for shame and embarrassment.

Many people suffering from tailbone pain and other pelvic pain syndromes unfortunately do feel embarrassed. You may feel awkward about discussing your pelvic symptoms and diagnosis, in a way that you would not feel awkward discussing similar problems at your shoulder or knee.

On a societal level, this needs to stop. We need to remove the old taboos that inhibit openly discussing pelvic problems.

We need to move the public discussion forward for tailbone pain. Far too many people unnecessarily suffer in silence because they feel awkward or embarrassed about discussing their tailbone pain. Do not let this be you. Empower yourself with knowledge and open

**Arming yourself with knowledge is a great defense against the frustrations and stigma of suffering with tailbone pain.**

communication. Make a positive difference for yourself and others who are affected by this condition. You can speak up for yourself and for others.

## What's Funny about Pain?

People without any tailbone pain sometimes think there's something funny about it. If a famous celebrity or politician suffered a fracture to their finger versus toe versus shoulder versus tailbone, which one of those would late night comedians poke fun at? It would be the tailbone.

It's not clear why some people consider the tailbone to be funny somehow. Perhaps it goes back to our early childhood days, when farts and such in that region seemed silly. Or perhaps the humor is just an adaptive mechanism for dealing with the awkwardness of discussing a topic of societal taboo.

Humor can be a terrific coping mechanism for someone who is suffering, but only if the person suffering is initiating or at least enjoying the humor. Many of my patients jokingly refer to their tailbone as being "a pain in the butt." But if their spouse, doctor, or neighbor joked about this in a callous way, it would be insensitive and hurtful. When it comes to joking about someone else's pain, it's best to follow the lead of the person who is actually suffering.

## Psychology, Depression, Anxiety

All pain and suffering includes an emotional experience. But it's crucial to point out that this is NOT saying that the emotional components are the cause of the pain. Far too many patients with coccydynia and other pelvic pains have their symptoms dismissed as "just due to emotional factors." Or the patient may be incorrectly told that the pain is "all in your head."

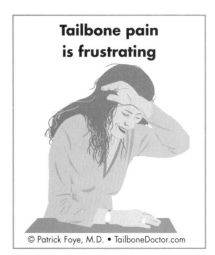

**Tailbone pain
is frustrating**

© Patrick Foye, M.D. • TailboneDoctor.com

Suffering from chronic daily pain for months and years is very draining, both physically and emotionally. Your pain can easily become the focus of your life, around which everything else revolves.

Your tailbone pain may prevent you from going out to a sit-down meal with your family and friends. Your tailbone pain may prevent you from going out to the movies, or a musical, or a dance recital. The severe pain while sitting may prevent you from taking a plane trip or long car ride to visit family or friends or to attend a special event. You may be unable to sit long enough to do your job or attend your school classes.

All of this can lead to feelings of isolation and loss. These are normal feelings in response to the situation. You may feel down, or blue. You may feel depressed. This is called a "reactive" depression. This means that the depression is a response, or reaction, to the situation.

While reactive depression is different than primary depression (which can occur independent of life circumstances), it still requires attention and care. Treatment of depression is beyond the focus of this book, but can include everything from talking to a supportive friend, to optimizing diet and exercise (which releases endorphins, our bodies' internal "feel good" chemicals), to professional psychology counseling sessions, to prescription antidepressant medications from your doctor.

In addition to causing depression, chronic pain can also cause anxiety. Tailbone pain can make you feel anxious about what's causing it, whether it will ever get better, and how this may affect the rest of your life. There's also the minute-by-minute anxiety of what chair you can sit in, how long you can sit, and whether you have your pain medications with you or not.

Chronic pain goes hand-in-hand with feeling depressed and anxious. You may also feel irritable, which can cause further stress in your relationships with family or friends. You may become more short-tempered, or less patient. These are normal responses.

You may feel that no one understands your situation or your pain. To others who see you, you don't look "sick" or "disabled" the way you would if you had your leg in a cast or your arm in a sling.

Openly discussing your mood and feelings with your family and treating physicians can be very helpful.

Meanwhile, arming yourself with knowledge is a great defense against the frustrations and stigma of suffering with tailbone pain. Knowledge is power and this book puts that power in your hands.

## Bias from Doctors

Countless patients have told me that their doctors laughed or chuckled when first hearing about their tailbone pain. Many patients felt offended, and rightfully so.

Doctors are often dismissive, as they minimize or trivialize your tailbone symptoms. This is due to physician ignorance and insensitivity.

The doctors' ignorance likely stems from never having learned much about tailbone pain. Pelvic pain syndromes often seem like a mysterious "black box" to most physicians, as they lack education and training in this area.

Gender issues may also arise. Often there is a male doctor telling a female patient that her tailbone pain is "all in her head." Instead of admitting that he lacks the knowledge and skills to help her, he may dismiss her symptoms as somehow not being deserving of the attentive care he would provide for pain at other body regions.

It's bad enough that chronic pain can cause depression and anxiety. But if you are not receiving adequate answers and medical care then not only will your physical pain be worse, but your emotional frustration will be worse too. If you are frustrated with your doctor's response, you can diplomatically but candidly let him/her know your concerns.

Keep searching until you find a healthcare provider with the knowledge, skills and compassion to provide you with the care that you need. You're worth it. You deserve it. Take the necessary actions to get the care and relief that you want. This book will empower you with knowledge so you can take whatever actions are needed to find the best medical care possible.

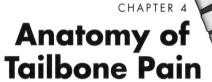

# CHAPTER 4

# Anatomy of Tailbone Pain

## Jessica's Story

As a graduate student in the visual arts, Jessica tried to picture in her mind what was causing her pain. She had heard that many people have low back pain, but she understood that low back pain was up around the waist line or belt line. Her pain was much lower down. But she did not know internal human anatomy well enough to know where the pain was coming from. So she searched online for images of back pain and buttock pain. Initially, most of the images were of the "lumbar" or "lumbosacral" spine. She could see that those images were showing areas higher than where she was having pain. Eventually, Jessica came across some images of the tailbone, at the lower end of the spine. She immediately knew that this was the site of her pain. She smiled with satisfaction at her successful discovery. Knowing the anatomy of where her pain was coming from was her first step in finding the underlying cause and the best possible treatment.

## Spinal Bones, Discs and Joints

The human spine is made up of a series of bones stacked one on top of the other. This spinal column extends from its uppermost part (just below the head/skull), down to its lower most part at the coccyx (in the buttocks region).

The spine is categorized into five distinct regions:
- the cervical spine (or neck),
- the thoracic spine (with attachments to the ribs),
- the lumbar spine (lower back region),
- the sacral spine (forming the sacrum, or back wall of the pelvis), and
- the coccygeal spine (tailbone).

Each of these regions has a typical number of spinal bones (also called vertebral bones) stacked on top of each other: 7 in the cervical spine, 12 in the thoracic spine, 5 in the lumbar spine, 5 in the sacral spine, and 3 to 5 in the coccygeal spine.

**The term "tailbone" incorrectly implies that it is a single bone.**

In between these spinal bones are the discs and spaces that help to absorb shock and other mechanical forces. There are also joints, which are sites where one bone meets (articulates) with another bone, often separated by a protective layer of cartilage.

The "sacrococcygeal joint" (or sacrococcygeal "junction") is located between the lowest sacral vertebral bone and the highest coccygeal vertebral bone. This junction includes the disc or cartilage that separates the fifth sacral bone from the first coccyx bone. Also, the sacrum has two bony projections that extend downward (the right and left sacral cornu, which means horns). While these sacral bony horns are extending downward toward the coccyx, there are corresponding coccygeal cornu (bony horn-like projections) extending up toward the sacrum. These articulations between the sacral cornu heading downward to meet the coccygeal cornu heading upward are referred to as the right and left sacrococcygeal facet joints (also called zygapophysial joints). The right and left sacrococcygeal facet (zygapophysial joints) are similar to the facet joints in the lumbosacral spine, which can also be sites of arthritis and pain.

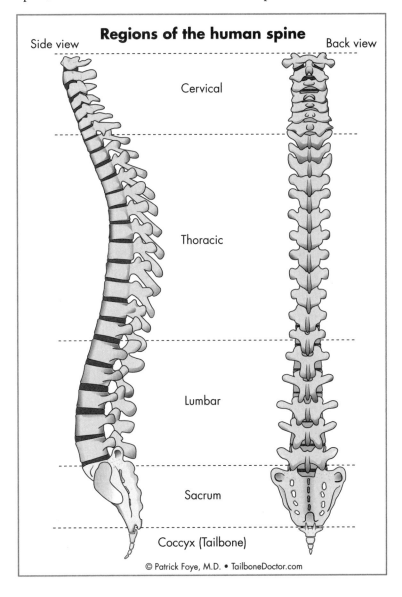

© Patrick Foye, M.D. • TailboneDoctor.com

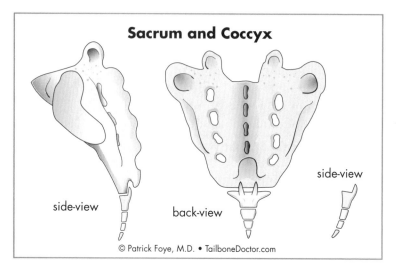

**Sacrum and Coccyx**

side-view   back-view   side-view

© Patrick Foye, M.D. • TailboneDoctor.com

## The Coccyx

As noted above, the coccyx is made of 3 to 5 spinal (vertebral) bones. No other region of the spine has this degree of variability in the number of bones present. This variability means that physicians cannot confidently know exactly what to expect before viewing x-rays, MRIs, or other medical images of your coccyx.

This variability can sometimes cause confusion or uncertainty, since radiologists, emergency room physicians, and other healthcare providers may see more bone segments than they expect and then incorrectly think that this is due to fracture. In fact, the number of bones present may just be your normal "baseline."

## Misnomer: Singular versus Plural

One roadblock to understanding anatomy of the coccyx is the misnomer of it being called the tailbone, or coccyx.

The term "tailbone" incorrectly implies that it is a single bone. So we have a series of 3 to 5 bones being referred to as a single bone. So, the term "tailbone" is misleading. It would be more accurate to refer to this as the tailboneS (plural), but no one does that. Similarly, the "coccyx" could be more descriptively called the "coccygeal bones" or "coccygeal vertebral segments," to emphasize that there is indeed a series of discrete bones, not just one singular item.

## Tailbone Function, Usefulness

Unlike many other primates, humans do not have actual tails. But we still have a few bony segments called the tailbone (coccyx). It's ignorant to say "humans don't have tails, so we don't need our tailbones." Your tailbone is an important attachment site for muscles, tendons, and ligaments of your pelvic floor. Knowing this protects you from incorrectly thinking that "since we don't have tails, the tailbone can be surgically removed with zero functional consequences."

As discussed in Chapter 2: *Symptoms of Tailbone Pain,* the tailbone also serves as a third (slight) weight bearing site while sitting, completing the midline part of the sit-bone triad or tripod (the other two sites being the right and left ischial bones).

## Looking Out for Number One

When looking at the coccyx in medical imaging studies such as x-rays (radiographs), MRI (magnetic resonance imaging), CT scans (computerized tomography scans), or fluoroscopy, it is extremely helpful to start by identifying the first (highest) coccygeal bone.

Only the first coccygeal bone has these two upward bony projections (cornu, or horns). Also, only this first coccygeal bone has the right and left sideways bony projections (transverse processes). The rest of the (lower) coccyx bones do not have either of these two features.

Easy ways to remember these two distinctive features of the first coccygeal bone are to think of an American football referee calling a field goal or a touchdown and separately think of a baseball umpire calling a runner safe at the plate.

When a football referee signals a field goal or a touchdown, he puts both arms up into the air, mimicking the two goalposts. Think of the referee as being the first coccygeal bone and his two arms reaching upward represent the right and left coccygeal cornu (which means horns). On imaging studies, the coccygeal bone that has these two upward projections is coccyx bone number one.

Mimicking a different part of coccyx bone number one, when a baseball umpire signals that the runner is "safe" at the plate, he extends both his arms out to each side. This could also be referred to as an airplane position, with the arms stretching out like airplane wings. On medical imaging studies if you see a coccygeal bone with these bony projections (transverse processes) extending outward to the right and left side, then you have specifically identified coccyx bone number one.

## Smaller Segments Lower Down

If you look at your index finger, you will notice that there are three bones of different lengths. As you move from the hand to the fingertip, each bone gets a little bit shorter and a little bit more slender. Similarly at the coccyx, as you move from the sacrum toward the lower tip of the tailbone, each of the coccygeal bones gets a little bit shorter and a little bit more slender.

Also, just as the joints in your index finger allow each bone to bend, or flex forward, so too do the coccygeal joints allow the coccygeal bones to flex forward.

When visualizing the tailbone it may be helpful for you to think of your index finger as representing the tailbone, with your hand representing the sacrum. (In reality, the sacrum is much bigger than your hand and the coccyx is smaller than your index finger, and even smaller than your pinky finger. But the hand and index finger comparison is easier for visualizing and demonstrating coccyx comparisons.)

## Muscle Attachments (Pelvic Floor)

The pelvic floor is a group of muscles, tendons and ligaments. The pelvic floor acts as a sling, or hammock, to support the pelvic organs and keep gravity from making them fall to the floor as we stand and walk.

Just as a hammock is attached at each end, the pelvic floor also has attachments to hold it in place and support it. At the back area of the pelvic floor, these attachments include the coccyx. Muscles and tendons that attach to the coccyx include:

- the right and left gluteus maximus muscles (the largest of the gluteal, or buttock muscles, active during walking),

- the coccygeus muscle, and

- the levator ani muscle group (which has three parts: the iliococcygeus muscle, the pubococcygeus muscle, and the puborectalis muscle).

### Ligaments

Ligaments that attach to the coccyx include:

- the anterior longitudinal ligament (along the front of the coccyx, where it is also known as the anterior sacrococcygeal ligament),

- the posterior sacrococcygeal ligament (along the back of the coccyx),

- the lateral sacrococcygeal ligament (attaching the sacrum to the right and left sides of the coccyx at the transverse processes of the first coccygeal bone),

- the spinosacral ligament (spanning from the right and left ischial spines to the sacrum and coccyx), and

- the sacrotuberous ligament (which attaches the sacrum and coccyx to the ischial tuberosity).

This collection of ligaments thus attach, span and cover the coccyx front and back, right and left, up and down, and on diagonals. The coccyx helps secure other bones in place, and vice versa.

## Nerves of the Coccyx

Just as there are nerves that carry pain and other sensations from the bones of your index finger, there are nerves that carry pain and other sensations from the bones of your coccyx. These are called "somatic" nerves. These somatic nerves at the coccyx carry pain upward, entering the sacral canal and from there traveling through the spine, upward to your brain.

The sympathetic nervous system has a final hub at the coccyx called the ganglion Impar. The nerve hub (ganglion) is involved in sympathetically-maintained pain (sympathetic nervous system pain) of the tailbone region. See Chapter 12: *Sympathetic Nervous System Pain at the Coccyx.*

## Summary

Knowledge of coccyx anatomy lays groundwork for understanding the causes, diagnostic tests and treatments of tailbone pain. The coccyx is the lowest section of the human spine, located just below the sacrum and above the anus. The coccyx contains 3 to 5 coccygeal bones, with attachments to many muscles, tendons, ligaments, and nerves. The coccyx is a useful and important attachment site for the pelvic bones and the pelvic floor muscles, tendons, and ligaments.

## Free Bonus for You

For your free handout showing detailed images and descriptions of tailbone anatomy, go to: **TailboneDoctor.com/forms**

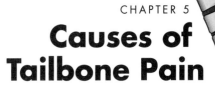

# CHAPTER 5

# Causes of Tailbone Pain

## Many Causes of Tailbone Pain

Yes, there are indeed many different causes of tailbone pain. The next several chapters will focus on causes of tailbone pain that are actually coming from the tailbone itself (rather than referred pain from other areas of the pelvis). So, these upcoming chapters will reveal a variety of painful tailbone conditions including fractures, dislocations, bone spurs, arthritis, unstable joints of the tailbone (dynamic instability), and many other causes.

The terms *coccydynia*, *coccyx pain*, *tailbone pain*, and *coccygodynia* all describe the underlying symptom of pain at the tailbone or tailbone region. But none of these terms explains what is causing the tailbone to be painful. Occasionally, the tailbone pain is "idiopathic" (a term meaning that the modern medical evaluation is unable to identify the specific cause). But a search for the specific cause of your tailbone pain is worthwhile and usually successful, if done properly. Knowing

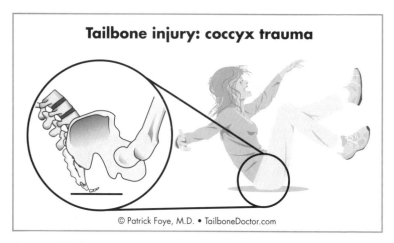

© Patrick Foye, M.D. • TailboneDoctor.com

the specific cause of your tailbone pain is important so that your treatment can be tailored to address what is causing your pain.

> **A search for the specific cause of your tailbone pain is worthwhile and usually successful, if done properly.**

Here is a list of many of the causes of tailbone pain, which you will discover in the next nine chapters in this book:

- Chapter 6: *Unstable Tailbone Joints: Dynamic Instability*
- Chapter 7: *Tailbone Fractures: The Broken Coccyx*
- Chapter 8: *Dislocations of the Tailbone*
- Chapter 9: *Bone Spurs of the Tailbone*
- Chapter 10: *Arthritis of the Tailbone*
- Chapter 11: *Abnormal Position of the Tailbone*
- Chapter 12: *Sympathetic Nervous System Pain at the Coccyx*
- Chapter 13: *Cancer Causing Tailbone Pain*
- Chapter 14: *Bone Infection Causing Tailbone Pain*

CHAPTER 6

# Unstable Tailbone Joints: Dynamic Instability

## Amanda's Story

Although Amanda understood why her tailbone pain was worse while sitting, she didn't understand why the pain skyrocketed during the few moments of going from sitting to standing. She dreaded getting up from a chair. Evaluation here at our Tailbone Pain Center revealed excessive looseness at her tailbone. This is one of the most common causes of tailbone pain. When Amanda sat, her tailbone went into a completely dislocated position. When she stood up, her tailbone would painfully snap back into normal alignment. After the few moments of pain from first standing up, it then felt fine while standing and walking (until the next time she sat down).

Her previous tailbone x-rays had only been done while standing, so they showed normal alignment of her coccyx (so she was incorrectly told that there was no cause for her pain). But Amanda's x-rays done while she was sitting showed the complete dislocation, confirming the diagnosis of coccygeal dynamic instability, which perfectly explained her tailbone pain. She had unstable joints in her tailbone. Fortunately, most people with this condition can be effectively treated without surgery.

## Unstable Tailbone Joints Causing Tailbone Pain

Unstable joints of the tailbone are probably the most under-appreciated, under-recognized, and under-diagnosed cause of tailbone pain. Unstable tailbone joints is a medical condition also called "coccygeal dynamic instability." This has been published in the medical literature since 1994, based on excellent innovation and research by Dr. Maigne. Unfortunately, most physicians, radiology technicians, and radiologists have still never heard of this diagnosis. In my

> **The coccyx often looks normal on those standard x-rays, because they failed to do the x-rays while you were sitting.**

practice evaluating hundreds of tailbone patients per year, unstable joints are found to be the underlying problem at least 20 times more commonly than tailbone fractures. Thus, understanding coccygeal dynamic instability is crucial since it is such a common and yet overlooked cause of tailbone pain.

## What Is Joint Instability at the Coccyx?

A joint is the site (or space) for connection and movement in between two bones. For every joint in the human body there is a normal, expected amount of movement. This normal amount of movement is what is seen in people who have no history of injury, pain or other problems at that joint.

An unstable joint is a joint that moves too much. Actually, you could describe an unstable joint either by saying that the "joint" moves too much, or by saying that the "bones" around the joint move too much. The position of the bone on one side of the joint

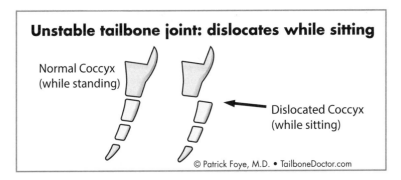

**Unstable tailbone joint: dislocates while sitting**

Normal Coccyx
(while standing)

Dislocated Coccyx
(while sitting)

© Patrick Foye, M.D. • TailboneDoctor.com

moves more than expected relative to the position of the bone on the other side of the joint.

## What Is "Dynamic" Instability?

Now that we understand what we mean by joint "instability," we now need to also understand what makes that instability "dynamic." Dynamic means that something is changing, that is, not fixed or static. So dynamic instability means that the appearance of the unstable joint changes. The bones of the joint may be in one position at one point in time and yet in a different position at another point in time.

Regarding dynamic instability specifically at the tailbone, the coccygeal bones may have normal positioning (alignment) while the patient is standing but have abnormal positioning (alignment) while the patient is sitting. In this way, the appearance of the joint (whether it looks stable or unstable) is "dynamic," or changing. This can partly explain why many patients with tailbone pain have little or no symptoms while they are standing up, but they may have severe pain while they are putting their body weight onto the tailbone by sitting.

## What Causes Joints to Be Unstable?

You can think of the coccygeal vertebral bones as being like a stack of bricks, stacked one on top of the other. The spaces between the bricks would represent the joint spaces between the bones. Duct tape from one brick to another would represent ligaments holding one bone to another. Just as a tear or rip in the duct tape would decrease the tape's ability to hold the bricks together, a tear in the coccygeal ligaments would decrease the ligaments' ability to hold the coccygeal bones together.

The coccygeal ligaments could be torn abruptly as a result of sudden direct, blunt trauma, such as falling onto the tailbone.

Alternatively, the ligaments could wear down gradually over the course of months and years. When this happens very gradually, patients start to develop instability even though they had no distinct or memorable episode of trauma. Similarly, you gradually wear down the brake pads in your car or the soles of your shoes over time even without a distinctly memorable incident of abnormal stress. Your coccygeal ligaments may gradually wear down over time without any distinct episode of coccygeal trauma.

## Different Movement Directions for the Unstable Tailbone

The different types of coccygeal dynamic instability are categorized based on the direction of the abnormal movement of the coccygeal bones. The bones may move excessively into flexion, or excessively into extension, or excessively out of alignment. Each of these types of instabilities will be addressed over the next few pages.

## "Flexion" Type of Coccygeal Dynamic Instability

You are already familiar with flexing and extending your elbow. Similarly, the coccygeal bones can flex and extend. If your arm is held straight, then flexing your elbow would be bringing the lower part of your arm and hand forward and upward toward your shoulder, such as when doing a biceps curl during weightlifting.

Conversely, extending your elbow would be straightening your arm back out, such that the lower portion of your arm and hand are moving downward and backward. So, there is a standard agreement for which direction is considered elbow flexion and which direction is considered elbow extension. The same is true at the coccyx.

"Flexion" at the coccyx refers to the lower portion of the coccyx (the lowest coccygeal bones) moving upward and forward. "Extension" at the coccyx refers to the lower portion of the coccyx moving downward and backward.

Coccygeal dynamic instability in the direction of flexion means that the amount of movement in the direction of flexion is more than normal. When most people sit down, this places some body weight onto the coccyx, which then tends to go into slight flexion. The lower coccyx moves slightly forward relative to the upper coccyx. This normal amount of forward flexion when sitting is measured as an angular movement, so it is measured in degrees. More specifically, it is measured as the change in degrees, meaning that the baseline angle of the coccyx while standing is compared with the angle of the coccyx while sitting. If the baseline angle of the tailbone while standing is 40 degrees of forward flexion but the angle of the tailbone while sitting is 50 degrees of forward flexion, then the change in degrees is the difference, which is 10 degrees. The normal amount of flexion movement when going from standing to sitting is less than 20 degrees of additional flexion (i.e., compared to the starting position while standing as per Dr. Maigne's 1994 article).

## "Extension" Type of Coccygeal Dynamic Instability

Extension is movement in the opposite direction to that of flexion. Back to our comparison, your elbow joints can flex (the lower part of your arm moves forward and upward) and extend (the lower part of our arm moves downward and backward). Similarly, your coccygeal joints can flex (lower coccygeal bones move forward and upward) and extend (lower coccygeal bones move downward and backward).

Coccygeal dynamic instability in the direction of extension, then, is when sitting causes the lower tailbone to move backward more than normal. This direction of movement is particularly problematic because the further the tailbone goes into extension the less protected it is, since it is no longer "tucked in" within the pelvis. So, while sitting, the weight-bearing onto the tailbone is increased if the tailbone is in a more extended position. This means that a joint that already has increased laxity and mobility is now subjected to even more physical stress because it is sticking out, that is, it's literally "in the way" of you sitting down.

## "Listhesis" Type of Coccygeal Dynamic Instability

"Listhesis" is the medical term for "sliding." Just as you can slide a drawer forward or backward (relative to the drawer above or below it), so too can the bones on either side of a joint slide slightly forward or backward (relative to the bone above or below it). When the coccygeal bones slide forward or backward relative to each other, they no longer have the optimal alignment of being stacked up neatly one on top of the other. A small amount of this type of movement during sitting is considered normal, but when it is excessive then this is coccygeal dynamic instability in listhesis.

Admittedly, the comparison to sliding a drawer back and forth is not a perfect comparison since a bureau (chest of drawers) has a back that prevents the drawer from sliding backward beyond its back wall. So imagine that the bureau has no backing on it, allowing the back-and-forth sliding to occur in either direction. With this modification, we have a more accurate comparison between the sliding bureau drawers and the sliding coccygeal bones.

Physicians measure and categorize listhesis based upon how much movement there has been of one bone relative to another. The measurement system for listhesis is based on the amount of sliding movement compared to the width (where bone width is the distance from the front of the bone to the back of the bone).

Let's come back to our bricks example. If the bricks are stacked perfectly one on top of the other, there is no listhesis. To keep the math simple, let's assume that each brick has a distance (or width) of four inches when measuring from the front of the brick to the back of the brick. If one brick moved forward by one inch, then it has moved forward by one-fourth (25 percent) of the brick's width. This would be 25 percent listhesis. If one brick moved forward or backward by two inches, then it has moved forward by two-fourths (50 percent) of the brick's width (50 percent listhesis). Similarly, forward movement by three inches would be three-fourths (75 percent listhesis). Forward movement by four inches would be four-fourths (100 percent listhesis). This 100 percent listhesis would mean that one brick has moved so much that it is no longer really in the stack at all. There would be no overlap with the next brick. By definition, this would be a 100 percent dislocation (100 percent listhesis).

Whether we are talking about a stack of bricks or a stack of coccygeal bones, the understanding of listhesis is the same. One coccygeal bone can slide (listhesis) forward or backward relative to the position of the coccygeal bone above or below it. The amount of listhesis is measured as a percentage, compared to the front-to-back width of the coccygeal bone.

The amount (percentage) of listhesis is grouped into categories described as Grade 1 through Grade 5. Specifically, listhesis is categorized as Grade 1 (1 to 25 percent listhesis), Grade 2 (26 to 50 percent listhesis), Grade 3 (51 to 75 percent listhesis), Grade 4 (76 to 100 percent listhesis), and Grade 5 (more than 100 pecent listhesis).

## "Joint Height Collapse" Type of Coccygeal Dynamic Instability

We have already discussed movement of the coccygeal bones into flexion and extension, as well as into listhesis (sliding forward and backward). But it is also possible for the coccygeal bones to move up and down.

Back to comparing the coccygeal bones to a stack of bricks, there are spaces between the bricks just as there are between coccygeal bones. The height of this space can be measured as the distance from the bottom of one brick to the top of the brick that is below it. If you saw a picture of a stack of bricks and noticed that there was an unusually tall space at the junction between one brick and the next brick, you may wisely guess that the stack is unstable at that junction. Similarly at the coccyx, an unusually tall joint space raises my suspicion that it is an unstable joint.

Further, when sitting puts weight-bearing stresses upon the coccyx, we would normally expect most of the joint height to be maintained. When there is an unusually tall coccygeal joint space, I am always interested to see what happens to that joint space during weight-bearing (sitting). Often, sitting causes dynamic instability at such a joint. As noted above, the instability might be excessive flexion or extension, or perhaps listhesis. But the instability could also be excessive movement in the up-and-down directions. During sitting, the body weight could push the bones closer together, decreasing the height of the joint space. When this movement is excessive, it is called "joint space collapse."

## Testing for Dynamic Instability

Dynamic x-rays (radiographs) are done to assess for coccygeal dynamic instability. Specifically, coccyx x-rays are done while the patient is sitting and also while he/she is standing (or lying down).

The coccyx is considered as "weight-bearing" during the seated x-rays and is considered "non-weight-bearing" during the standing x-rays. The position of the coccygeal bones while sitting is compared to the position while standing. A small amount of movement between the bones is considered normal, but excessive movement is considered abnormal (dynamic instability).

### How Much Movement Is "Normal"?

In the direction of flexion, a change in angle by *20 degrees* or more is considered abnormal.

For listhesis, movement by more than *25 percent* (of the coccygeal bone width) is considered abnormal.

For joint space collapse, we unfortunately do not have published research data to draw a specific cutoff between normal and abnormal movement. As a general rule of thumb in my practice, I consider joint collapse of more than *50 percent* (of the joint space height) to be abnormal.

### Where Can You Get Sitting versus Standing Coccyx X-rays Done?

Obtaining sit-stand x-rays is a huge challenge for patients and their doctors. Very few radiology centers have ever even heard of tailbone x-rays being done while you are sitting. Even if you go to your local radiology center and bring with them copies of medical journal articles or other materials explaining how the x-rays are done, you will likely be told that they cannot be done. Sometimes a radiology center will give it a try, but they lack experience from never having done this test before. This can result in the test being done incorrectly and thus failing to give you reliable results. Even if the radiology technician performs the test properly, the radiologist (the physician who reads your x-rays) has likely never heard of sitting-versus-standing coccyx x-rays and therefore may be unable to confidently read or interpret your x-rays.

This situation is extremely unfortunate, since coccygeal dynamic instability is the most common cause of tailbone pain. This means that for many people with tailbone pain their local radiology centers are unable to provide the optimal diagnostic tests to help reveal what is causing the pain. Typically, routine (old-fashioned) coccyx x-rays are done only while standing or lying down (not while sitting). The coccyx often looks normal on those standard x-rays, because they failed to do the x-rays while you were sitting. Then, you and your treating physician are told that there is no explanation for your pain. I see hundreds of patients each year where this exact scenario has occurred. The patients had been told there is no reason for their pain but in reality the optimal test to diagnose the cause had simply not been done yet.

Even in an academic setting such as mine at Rutgers New Jersey Medical School, it was an uphill battle for me to have our own radiology department start providing these sitting-versus-standing x-rays. Initially, I had to personally walk each of my tailbone patients down to radiology and direct the radiology technicians on how to properly perform these x-rays. I needed to do this for many months, along with providing in-service training sessions for the radiology technicians. The benefits were well worth it, as they became competent and reliable at performing these sitting-versus-standing x-rays properly, leading to successful diagnosis for patients who come from around the world.

I have often tried to help people far away to obtain these studies at their local hospitals or radiology centers, by speaking with physicians, radiology technicians, and radiologists. But it is nearly impossible to successfully do this, and the initial attempts at any given facility tend to be of poor quality and thus limited usefulness.

In the United States, many patients travel to see me in New Jersey where my evaluation for tailbone pain almost always includes doing these sitting-versus-standing x-rays. Using these images, we can usually discover the underlying cause of the tailbone pain. I also continue working to educate physicians through medical publications and conferences, but so far it has been an uphill battle.

## Treatments for Coccygeal Dynamic Instability

The available treatments are discussed in Chapters 18 through 25. Overall, treatments include avoiding things that make your pain worse (Chapter 19), trying various tailbone cushions (Chapter 20), using medications (Chapter 21), and undergoing small local injections (Chapter 24). In the rare cases where these treatments are not helpful, you may even consider surgical removal of the coccyx (Chapter 25), but only after a valid attempt to get relief through non-surgical options.

### Free Bonus for You

For your free handout showing and describing unstable joints of the tailbone, including details on performing and evaluating sitting x-rays of the tailbone, go to: **TailboneDoctor.com/forms**

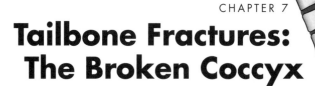

# CHAPTER 7

# Tailbone Fractures: The Broken Coccyx

## Michael's Story

While getting out of his delivery truck, Michael slipped and fell. His tailbone landed hard against the road. Although initial x-rays failed to detect any fracture, he suffered in pain for months. Eventually, better imaging tests later revealed that he had shattered his tailbone into pieces. Years earlier he had fractured his forearm and it had been promptly and easily diagnosed. By comparison, why had the initial coccyx x-rays missed his fracture? His forearm fracture had been treated with a cast and a sling. Now Michael wondered if there was any way to get a cast or a sling for his fractured tailbone. Also, his forearm fracture had been pain-free within several weeks. Why was his tailbone fracture still so painful for so many months? He wondered why tailbone fractures are so much more difficult to diagnosis and treat than most fractures elsewhere in the body.

**Tailbone fractures are more challenging than fractures in other body regions.**

## What Is a Tailbone Fracture?

A fracture is commonly known as a broken bone. This means that the bone has lost its normal, relatively solid, intact form. There are many different types of fractures that can occur.

Sometimes a small chip will break off from the rest of the bone. Even if this chip of bone is tiny, the fracture itself can be very painful and problematic. Further, the chip of bone may enter the joint space, disrupting normal movement of the joint and tearing the cartilage within the joint.

In other cases, the break may just be a "hairline fracture," which is a crack within the bone but without any piece of the bone that separates from the rest of the bone. I often compare hairline fractures to having a crack within a sheetrock wall

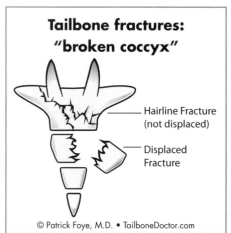

**Tailbone fractures: "broken coccyx"**

Hairline Fracture (not displaced)

Displaced Fracture

© Patrick Foye, M.D. • TailboneDoctor.com

or within the concrete foundation for a house. Even though no piece of the wall or foundation has come off, the crack represents an injury and a lack of integrity of the structure.

In other cases, the patient may have a "compression" fracture, where the bone is compressed (crushed down upon itself). I often explain a compression fracture as being like crushing a Styrofoam cup. Even if no piece of the cup separates from the rest, the crushed cup overall is deformed.

Lastly, in some cases a coccygeal bone can be completely shattered into many pieces. This is called a "comminuted" fracture.

In summary, there are multiple types of fractures that can occur at the coccyx. And not surprisingly, a fractured bone causes pain.

## How Does a Tailbone Fracture Happen?

A fracture is usually caused by sudden trauma or injury. For example, you may slip and fall, landing directly on your tailbone. Your tailbone is vulnerable to traumatic injuries for multiple reasons.

First, there is no substantial "padding" behind or below the tailbone. Although we humans have substantial gluteal muscle tissue providing padding at each buttock (right and left), there is no such muscle tissue providing padding behind the tailbone. This means that the forces of blunt trauma to the tailbone region are delivered more directly and more forcefully, causing tailbone injury.

Another reason why your tailbone may be vulnerable to injury during a fall could be the pre-existing, baseline anatomy of the tailbone. For example, a patient without any symptoms might have a tailbone that extends slightly backward (instead of the normal tailbone angle, which is forward). When this person falls, their tailbone is sticking slightly backward (outward) where it will be injured (rather than being in the normal position safely flexed slightly forward into the pelvis, where it would be more protected from such an *external* trauma).

Alternatively, a patient may have a tailbone that is flexed too far forward into the pelvis, where it may experience *internal* trauma. For example, when a baby is being born through that birth canal, the internal pressure onto the excessively-forward coccyx can cause tailbone injury. (See Chapter 27: *Pregnancy, Childbirth and Tailbone Pain.*) Sometimes even the forces and pressure from a bowel movement (stool moving through the rectum) may cause pressure onto the excessively-forward coccyx, thus causing tailbone pain.

In some cases, the pre-existing problem is not so much the position of the tailbone but the lack of flexibility of the tailbone. The patient may have a tailbone that is too stiff, lacking sufficient movement at the joints between the coccygeal bones. The stiff tailbone lacks the flexibility to move or bend in response to the abrupt external trauma of a fall to the floor. If the force delivered to the coccygeal bones is greater than the strength of the bones to resist such force, a fracture may occur. Note that a tailbone that is too stiff can be fractured due to either *external* forces (such as falling, with the tailbone hitting the floor) or *internal* forces (such as a baby passing through the birth canal).

## How Is a Tailbone Fracture Diagnosed?

Medical imaging studies are needed to confirm a diagnosis of tailbone fracture. These imaging studies can include x-rays, CT scans and MRIs. These and other tests will be discussed in more detail in Chapter 16: *Medical Tests for Tailbone Pain*.

## Challenging Symptoms and Physical Exam Findings

In many ways, tailbone fractures are more challenging than fractures in other body regions. It can be more difficult for physicians to diagnose a tailbone fracture than it is for many other types of fractures. The coccygeal bones are small and are flexed forward (tucking themselves partway into the pelvis), so fractures of these bones rarely cause the kind of blatantly obvious bruising and swelling that is often seen with many fractures of the arms, legs or face.

Further, many patients have less "body awareness" for their pelvic anatomy than they do for other parts of the body. This means that a patient who fractures his toe or thumb would present to the physician already being able to accurately specify which body site was injured. But at the tailbone most patients would be much less certain. Ideally, the patient would go to a physician experienced at evaluating injuries in the tailbone region. But, unfortunately, many physicians have little or no training, experience or competence at properly evaluating tailbone injuries. Doctors may be uncertain or inexperienced regarding how to perform a proper physical examination of the tailbone. This combination of factors can make the history and physical exam problematic in the evaluation of a tailbone fracture.

## Proper Imaging Studies to Diagnose a Tailbone Fracture

Doctors may be uncertain or inexperienced regarding how to order the appropriate diagnostic tests to assess tailbone injuries. Even if the physician orders the imaging studies (such as x-rays or MRI or CT scans) properly, the radiology technician may be uncertain or inexperienced regarding how to properly perform the requested tests. And even if the radiology technician does perform the imaging studies properly, many radiologists (physicians who specialize in reading the images) may be uncertain or inexperienced regarding how to properly evaluate the appearance of the tailbone.

Regarding these physicians, radiology technicians, and radiologists, most of them are wonderful people and are terrific, caring, dedicated, and smart healthcare professionals. It really just comes down to experience. Physicians with limited experience or training regarding a specific condition may provide less clinical excellence than they would for conditions that they see more often.

The bottom line: tailbone injuries are uncommon enough that many physicians and radiology technicians do not see them frequently enough to develop adequate evaluation skills and treatment expertise.

## Number of Coccygeal Bones, Pieces

The number of coccygeal bones creates yet another fairly unique challenge when it comes to evaluating for coccyx fractures. Specifically, since there is a baseline of high variability in the number of coccygeal bony segments (coccygeal vertebral bones), this can make it difficult for physicians to assess whether there has been a fracture that has resulted in an additional piece of bone having broken off. In other body sites, if you see an extra piece of bone you can immediately suspect that it is a fracture. But the baseline variability in the number of coccygeal bones even prior to fracture makes it more difficult to know whether there is an "extra" bone due to fracture (rather than being just the normal baseline number of bones for that specific patient).

The very terminology of calling it a "tailbone" is misleading and can mentally lead a physician to an incorrect diagnosis. Specifically, the term "tailbone" is singular, implying that there is a single bone at this body region. Nobody refers to it as the "tailbone*S*," even though that would be more accurate, since the plural term tailbone*S* would clearly designate that there are multiple bone*S* making up what is typically (misleadingly) called the "tailbone." Similarly, a tailbone is often referred to as a coccyx, which is again a singular term incorrectly implying that it is just one bone. It would be less misleading to instead refer to it as the "coccygeal bones."

The singular versus plural terminology for tailbone and coccyx is clinically important in understanding coccyx fractures. A physician must understand the normal number of coccygeal bones before being able to analyze whether there is an abnormal number of coccygeal bones. An emergency room physician may declare that you have a fractured tailbone, when in actuality the physician just noticed that there were multiple coccygeal bones (plural), and since it was more than one piece of bone the physician thus incorrectly assumed that it must have been a fracture (that is, he was thinking it was originally a single bone that had fractured into the two or three pieces).

## Treatment of a Tailbone Fracture

After diagnosis, fractures at most sites in the body are treated by immobilization (decreasing the bony movement at the fracture site) and limiting the weight-bearing, use, or other stresses upon the fracture. But at the tailbone, all of these treatment approaches are limited or impossible.

Immobilizing a fracture or joint prevents it from moving. Immobilization helps allow the injured site to heal. Fractures repair themselves by mending or bridging bone across the fracture site. Repetitive movement across the fracture site makes it difficult or impossible for the fracture to heal.

Immobilization is practically impossible at the site of a coccygeal fracture. A broken arm or leg could be placed into a solid cast to prevent movement at the fracture site. But there is no similar way to put a cast across the coccyx.

A broken arm or leg could be treated by surgically placing a metal plate across the fracture site. The plate is screwed into the bone above and below the site of the fracture, to ensure that no movement occurs at the fracture site (thus immobilizing the fracture so that it can heal). But the bones of the coccyx are very small and would not tolerate having screws drilled into them. Also, many patients with tailbone pain already report that they feel like they are sitting on something sharp or pointy. Placing screws, rods, or orthopedic hardware plates onto or into the coccyx would most likely make the pain worse. This could be problematic especially when the patient is sitting, since while sitting the patient would be putting body weight onto the screws and plates. So, coccyx fractures really cannot be immobilized.

Aside from immobilization, fractures at other body sites are often treated by limiting weight-bearing on the fracture site. If someone has a fractured leg, the person can use crutches to move around without putting any body weight onto that leg. If someone has a fractured arm, they can avoid pushing and lifting with that arm, to avoid causing any weight to stress at the fracture site.

But at the tailbone, weight-bearing happens with sitting, and sitting is very difficult to avoid. Most people do not have the endurance to spend the entire day standing up. Nor do most people have a bed or couch to lie down on while at work. Sitting is a pervasive activity in modern society. We sit when we attend classes, conferences and meetings. We sit when we use our computers, drive our cars, eat our meals, watch television, or chat with a friend. So, it would be very challenging for someone with a coccyx fracture to avoid weight-bearing at the fracture site, since he/she would essentially need to avoid all sitting, for many weeks, to allow the fracture to heal.

Lastly, even if someone could avoid sitting (and thus avoid weight-bearing on the coccyx), other stresses at the fracture site would continue. Even just the simple act of walking can place some mechanical stresses on the coccyx, since some of the gluteal (buttock) muscles and pelvic floor muscles attach directly to the coccyx.

In summary, coccyx fractures present unique challenges since it is difficult (probably impossible) to limit fracture movement and weight-bearing in the way that those typically would be limited in treating fractures at other body regions.

### How Common Are Coccyx Fractures?

Coccyx fractures are much less common than coccyx dislocations and coccygeal "dynamic instability," all of which will be discussed in detail within other chapters of this book. (See Chapter 6: *Unstable Tailbone Joints: Dynamic Instability.* Also see Chapter 8: *Dislocations of the Tailbone.*)

### Free Bonus for You

For your free printable handout showing and describing risks and categories for tailbone fractures, go to: **TailboneDoctor.com/forms**

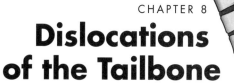

# CHAPTER 8

# Dislocations
# of the Tailbone

## Kimberly's Story

Kimberly was having blast on summer vacation with her family.
They loved trips where they could enjoy "fun in the sun"
activities. She was riding a jet ski when, unfortunately, her
tailbone hit hard against the seat while she sped across
choppy, bumpy waves. She had immediate pain that took
her breath away. She spent that night of her vacation in
the local emergency room, where they told her she would
feel fine within a few weeks. But two years later, her
tailbone pain was still severe. Our x-rays revealed that
she had a complete, 100 percent dislocation at one
of the joints within her tailbone. The bones at each
side of that joint were completely out of alignment.
By focusing our treatment to that one specific joint,
she finally obtained complete relief.

## What Is a Dislocation?

A joint is the site where two or more bones interact or
articulate with each other. A dislocation is when a bone at

either side of a joint moves out of its normal position. For example, one bone may move too far forward relative to the position of the bone at the other side of a joint space. The bone that has moved into an abnormal position is referred to as being a dislocated bone. The involved joint is referred to as a dislocated joint.

## Dislocation versus Fracture

As previously discussed in the chapter on tailbone fractures, a fracture is when there is a break within the substance of the bone itself. (See Chapter 7: *Tailbone Fractures: The Broken Coccyx*.) This break within the bone is different from a dislocation. Unlike a fracture, a dislocation retains normal integrity of the bone itself, but the joint *in between* the bones is compromised.

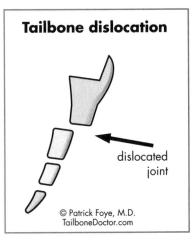

**Tailbone dislocation**

dislocated joint

© Patrick Foye, M.D.
TailboneDoctor.com

As a comparison, simply think of a stack of three bricks, one on top of the other. The bricks would represent the bones and the spaces in between the bricks would represent the joints. If some trauma forcefully caused one of the bricks to be broken, that would be equivalent to a fracture. Alternatively, if the forces left all the bricks intact (unbroken), but knocked one of the bricks off the stack, that would be a dislocation. Thus, if there is no chip or crack in the brick (or bone) then it is not a fracture. Dislocation, then, refers to the abnormal position or misalignment of the bricks (bones).

**Multiple factors make it difficult to accurately and confidently diagnose a tailbone dislocation.**

The bricks offer a simplistic explanation. But it provides a great starting point for understanding the differences between tailbone fractures and dislocations. I have seen many cases where physicians have confused and collapsed these terms when evaluating medical imaging of the tailbone, when they would not make such errors at other body regions.

## Ligaments Involved in Tailbone Dislocations

Ligaments are strong but flexible connective tissue structures that attach one bone to another bone. A ligament attaches a bone to a bone, whereas a tendon attaches a muscle to a bone.

There are several ligaments at the coccyx, creating a balance between flexibility and stability. Along the front of the coccyx is the anterior longitudinal ligament (which here is also called the anterior sacrococcygeal ligament). Along the back of the coccyx is the posterior longitudinal ligament. There are other ligaments as well.

Back to our comparison of the coccygeal bones being like a stack of bricks. If we used duct tape to bind the stack together, then the ligaments would be like the duct tape spanning from one brick to the next, helping to hold those bricks in place. If the duct tape was torn then it would allow more movement between the bricks, just as a ligament being torn would allow more movement between the bones.

## What Challenges Are There in Diagnosing a Dislocation Specifically at the Tailbone?

Many factors make it difficult to accurately and confidently diagnose a tailbone dislocation.

First, since almost no one has baseline images of his/her tailbone before the start of having pain symptoms, we therefore do not know the exact baseline (prior to pain) position or alignment of the tail-bone for that specific person. To diagnose that a bone has moved out of its typical position, ideally we need to know what the baseline position was. Fortunately, even without such previous images to use as a reference, we can still often diagnosis a dislocation. If the dislocation is substantial or severe, we can readily detect that even without having previous baseline images to compare to. But if the dislocation is more mild or subtle, detecting it can be challenging.

A second challenge is that a certain amount of movement is normal at most joints. So, when evaluating whether a joint is dislo-cated the question is not whether there has been "any" movement at the joint, but instead the question is whether there has been "too much" movement at the joint.

The third challenge in evaluating for tailbone dislocations is that we humans have so much variability in our tailbones. As a baseline, from one person to the next, we have significant variability in the number of coccygeal bones we have, the position or alignment of those coccygeal bones, and the amount of movement at the joints between those coccygeal bones. This variability makes it even tougher to confidently say what the previous bone and joint posi-tions were prior to pain or injury. Without such baseline reference points it can be tough, but fortunately not impossible, to say if something has changed.

## Symptoms and Physical Exam Findings

Patients and physicians may have less certainty regarding dislocations at the coccygeal bones, compared with dislocations at other body regions. The reasons are similar to those previously discussed in the chapter on tailbone fractures. (See Chapter 7: *Tailbone Fractures: The Broken Coccyx*.) For example, if you dislocated your thumb or shoulder then you and your doctor would generally know that it was your thumb or shoulder. But if you dislocated a coccygeal bone neither you nor your doctor can directly see the coccyx dislocation with the naked eye.

## Medical Diagnostic Tests

Dislocations at the coccyx are diagnosed by looking at medical imaging tests, such as x-rays, CT scans (computerized tomography scans), or MRIs (magnetic resonance imaging). X-rays are the least expensive and most readily available, so x-rays are typically the first line tests. However, CT scans or MRIs may be helpful and even medically necessary in some individual cases. The pluses and minuses of the different imaging studies will be discussed in detail within Chapter 16: *Medical Tests for Tailbone Pain.*

## Treatment of Dislocations at Other (Non-coccyx) Body Regions

In most parts of the body, a dislocated bone is treated by placing the bone back into its normal position (by "relocating" the dislocated bone) followed by somehow then holding the bone in that normal position (immobilization). For example, a dislocated thumb would be put back into normal alignment and then an orthopedic cast would be placed to hold it that way while healing takes place. Similarly, a dislocated shoulder would be relocated back into its normal position and then that arm would be kept in a sling for some time to decrease further movement as the joint starts to heal. In cases where temporary casts and slings are not enough to restore joint integrity, surgery can be performed to tighten up the joint capsule, ligaments, or other anatomic structures. Surgical hardware, such as plates and screws, can be used to span and stabilize the dislocating joint.

## Challenges and Differences Treating a Dislocation at the Coccyx

As discussed in Chapter 7: *Tailbone Fractures: The Broken Coccyx*, it is simply not possible to immobilize the coccygeal bones the way that we can immobilize most other body regions. There is no coccyx cast or sling to use. Also, the small coccygeal bones and their location (weight-bearing onto them while sitting) means that they are not well suited for orthopedic hardware like plates and screws.

## Does That Mean That There Is No Treatment Available for a Tailbone Dislocation?

No. The good news is that treatments are indeed available for tailbone dislocations. But it's important to understand that the treatments are not the same as they would be for dislocations in other areas. A wide variety of treatments will be discussed in detail in Chapters 18 through 25.

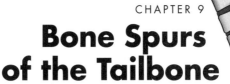

# CHAPTER 9

# Bone Spurs of the Tailbone

## Michelle's Story

Michelle had no history of trauma to her tailbone, so her pain there came out of the blue. It gradually became more and more painful. When she put her finger on the skin over the most painful spot she could feel a hard bump at the lower tip of her tailbone. Regular coccyx x-rays were too hazy or washed-out to clearly show the lower tip of her tailbone, thus failing to adequately show the spot where Michelle was having her pain. Coned-down x-rays here at our Tailbone Pain Center revealed an obvious bone spur at that exact spot. We looked at the x-rays together and she said, "Wow! That's exactly what it feels like." Michelle was relieved to finally have an answer that made sense. She was even more relieved to learn that coccyx bone spurs can usually be successfully treated without surgery.

## What Is a Bone Spur?

A bone spur is additional bone extending or projecting out from the normal bone. A bone spur is where the bone has become

**Tailbone bone spurs are typically located at the lowest point of the tailbone.**

bigger than normal, in a focal (localized) extension that often comes to a point. A bone spur is like an icicle extending down from a frozen rain gutter. The frozen rain gutter would represent the normal bone and the icicle extending (or projecting) down would represent the bone spur.

## What Is the Bone Spur Made Of? How Does It Form?

The bone spur is made of bone. It is bone. In most ways it's similar to the rest of the bone that it extends from. The main difference is that the spur is an extension or projection of bone beyond the typical, normal edges of the bone.

A bone spur is created when additional bone is formed in a focal location extending beyond the normal borders of the bone. By comparison, in other body regions we know that *skin* will gradually thicken and form into a callous in response to repetitive stresses (such as manual labor or walking barefoot). Similarly, *bone* may gradually thicken and form into a bone spur in response to repetitive stresses upon the bone (such as repeated weight-bearing onto the coccyx while sitting).

## Where Along the Coccyx Do Most Bone Spurs Occur?

Although theoretically a bone spur could happen at any location on bones, in actuality we see characteristic, specific body locations where bone spurs occur most commonly. For example, many people with shoulder pain have a bone spur indenting into their rotator cuff muscles. The bone spur at the shoulder often causes pain when the person tries to raise their arm overhead. Many people with foot pain have a bone spur at the sole of their foot, extending from the heel bone (a heel spur). A heel spur causes pain when patients put their body weight onto that foot during walking.

Similarly, many people with tailbone pain have a bone spur at the tailbone. Tailbone bone spurs are typically located at the lowest point of the tailbone. A coccyx bone spur causes pain when you are sitting, which puts pressure on the spur.

## In What Direction Do Most Coccyx Bone Spurs Extend?

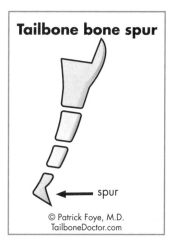

**Tailbone bone spur**

spur

© Patrick Foye, M.D.
TailboneDoctor.com

From the lowest end of the coccyx, bone spurs typically extend downward and backward. This is in direct contrast to the normal angle of the coccyx, where normally the lower parts of the tailbone flex forward into the pelvis.

## How a Bone Spur Causes Coccyx Pain

When bone extends beyond its normal and typical location, it can press on other nearby anatomic tissues or structures. So, a bone spur causes pressure onto nearby areas. Similarly, those adjacent areas can cause pressure back onto the bone spur. Since bone and other human tissue are innervated by nerves that carry pain, this abnormal pressure causes pain to the patient.

The normal tailbone position is flexed forward and therefore is tucked into the pelvis. Thus, the tailbone is somewhat protected and out-of-the-way when someone is sitting down. But when a patient has a bone spur extending in the opposite direction (backward instead of forward), then this bone spur is *not* tucked out-of-the-way. Instead the coccygeal bone spur is directly "in-the-way" of where you want to sit. Unlike the normal coccyx, which only mildly supports your body weight, a coccygeal bone spur causes the tailbone to support more of your body weight, which causes more tailbone pain. The spur extending downward and backward from the lower coccyx causes the tailbone to make more substantial contact with the chair or other sitting surface, resulting in increased weight-bearing forces being placed onto the coccyx. Also, the pointy lower end of the bone spur can pinch the skin in between the chair and the pointed lowest tip of the bone spur, increasing the pain even further.

## Sitting Positions That Worsen Bone Spur Pain

As with most other causes of tailbone pain, coccygeal bone spurs are most painful when you sit leaning partly backward, in a slightly reclining position. Since the bone spur typically extends downward and backward from the lower tip of the coccyx, sitting leaning partly backward painfully worsens how much the spur pinches the skin against the chair.

## Diagnosing a Bone Spur

Sometimes a bone spur is so prominent that it can be very clearly felt during a careful physical exam. This is done by the physician (or even by the patient herself/himself) pressing a fingertip against the back of the coccyx and "walking" it down to the lowest tip of the coccyx. A substantial bone spur may be felt projecting backward from the lower coccyx.

More commonly, a bone spur is diagnosed by looking at specific medical imaging studies such as x-rays, MRI, or CT scans. On medical imaging studies, a bone spur is best seen when looking at the coccyx from the side. For x-rays this is called the "lateral" view, whereas on MRI and CT scans this is called the "sagittal" view. These views allow you to see the normal forward-sloping curve or angle of the sacrum and coccyx, as well as abnormalities such as the exact opposite curve (the reverse angle) of the backward-sloping lower coccygeal bone spur.

## Bone Spur Size

I have seen hundreds of patients with coccygeal bone spurs and the size of the spur does not predict the severity of the pain. Many patients have been told by their local treating physician that the bone spur shown on imaging studies is too small to be of any concern, or too small to cause any pain or other symptoms. But on physical examination I often find that the exact site of severe, focal tenderness to palpation (pressing with my fingertip) is exactly localized to the bone spur seen on the imaging studies. The cause of pain is clear, even if the spur size was small!

I compare this to having a small pebble in your shoe. A pebble the size of a coccygeal bone spur may not seem like much. But walking around with your body weight pressing down onto that pebble would cause foot pain. Similarly, even a small coccygeal bone spur can be painful when you are sitting and thus putting your body weight onto that spur.

## Can You Surgically Shave Off the Bone Spur?

The answer is no. Although in other body regions bone spurs can indeed be surgically shaved down, this is not a typical treatment at the coccyx. The coccyx is a weight-bearing site (while sitting) and therefore just shaving down the lowest tip of the coccyx would cause there to be weight-bearing onto an area of raw, cut bone. Ouch! If a bone spur truly is to be surgically removed, the surgical approach is usually to remove not just the spur, but instead to remove the entire coccyx (coccygectomy). But this would be like amputating your finger as a treatment for a hangnail. Yes, it would remove the problem, but it is clearly more drastic than necessary.

However, the good news is that coccygeal bone spurs do tend to respond well to other forms of treatment, including nonsurgical treatments such as medications by mouth, cushions, and various pain management injections. All of these are discussed in significant details in Chapters 18 through 25, so keep reading.

## Free Bonus for You

For your free printable step-by-step guide to recognizing and diagnosing coccyx bone spurs, go to: **TailboneDoctor.com/forms**

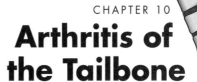

# CHAPTER 10

# Arthritis of the Tailbone

## David's Story

David had an aching soreness at his tailbone whenever he was sitting. He had never fallen onto it or had other blunt trauma there. He did have a history of arthritis in his knees, hips, and lower back. So he was not surprised when our evaluation revealed that he also had arthritis at his tailbone.

## What Is Arthritis?

The word arthritis refers to an abnormality of a joint, which is the site where two or more bones meet. The ending "-itis" refers to inflammation. Arthritis can be associated with excessive inflammation at the involved joint.

## Different Types of Arthritis

There are many different types of arthritis. The most common is osteoarthritis, which is a "degenerative" or "wear-and-tear" type of arthritis. This means that the bones and joint lining wear down over time. For example, knee joints and hip joints develop osteoarthritis after decades of normal weight-bearing activities such as standing and walking. Similarly, coccygeal joints can develop osteoarthritis after decades of normal weight-bearing activities such as sitting.

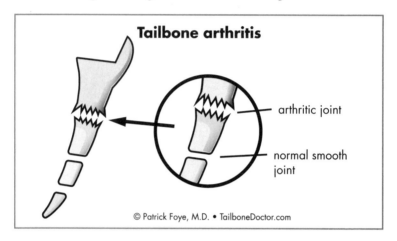

## Trauma Causing Arthritis

Trauma to bones and joints can be either gradual or sudden. Gradual repetitive trauma at your coccyx would be the normal forces from decades of coccygeal weight-bearing while sitting. Alternatively, sudden, abrupt trauma can occur. For example, you may have fallen directly onto your tailbone. Aside from the short-term pain and injury, the abrupt trauma may set the stage for developing post-traumatic arthritis at the involved joints years later.

## How Is Arthritis Diagnosed?

Arthritis is generally diagnosed by looking at medical imaging studies, such as x-rays, MRIs, or CT scans. On these imaging studies, instead of the normal bony borders of the joint space looking crisp, clean, and smooth, they may instead appear irregular or fuzzy. The bone at one or both sides of the joint may start to extend sideways beyond its normal borders, due to excess growth of bone. This extra bone is often called an "osteophyte" or "osteophytic lipping."

## Arthritis Causes Pain

Arthritis causes pain in several ways. First, arthritis is typically associated with inflammation of the joint, and your body's inflammatory chemicals can cause pain at the site of inflammation.

Second, arthritis can worsen to the point where the joint space is completely worn down. So rather than the cartilage or disc within the joint space helping to make a smooth articulation between one bone and the next bone, instead you may have "bone-on-bone." This means that one bone is contacting or rubbing against the bone above or below it. Because bones have nerve endings, this bone-rubbing-bone situation is painful.

**Coccygeal joints can develop osteoarthritis after decades of normal weightbearing activities such as sitting.**

Third, arthritis often causes stiffness within the joint. The coccygeal joints need to be able to bend slightly forward when we sit, to prevent the bones from contacting the chair. When stiff joints prevent the bones from moving out-of-the-way, the bones fail to move into the protected position of being tucked into the pelvis. The unprotected coccygeal bones then make more contact with the seat, resulting in more weight-bearing and more pain.

## Treatments for Tailbone Arthritis

Treatments are covered extensively in upcoming chapters. In general, these include avoiding exacerbating factors (Chapter 19), using tailbone cushions (Chapter 20), using medications topically or by mouth (Chapter 21), using medications given by small local injections (Chapter 24), and in very rare cases surgical removal of the coccyx (coccygectomy, discussed in Chapter 25).

CHAPTER 11

# Abnormal Position of the Tailbone

## Amy's Story

Amy wasn't sure whether her pain was being caused by a tailbone problem or a rectal problem. Her pain was worse right before and during bowel movements. She had consulted a gastroenterologist and he had even performed a colonoscopy, only to reveal that the insides of her rectum and colon appeared normal, without any visible cause for her symptoms. Amy had also undergone x-rays and an MRI, and again she was told that her results were normal. So many tests, yet still no answers. But she brought the images to her initial evaluation here at the Tailbone Pain Center. Closer inspection revealed that her tailbone was abruptly flexing forward and actually indenting into the wall of the rectum (where stool is stored before a bowel movement). This perfectly explained her symptoms. Finally, Amy had an answer.

Sometimes the tailbone is in an abnormal position. Variability from person to person means that the curve, or angle, of your tailbone can be different than someone else's.

This variability may be minor and cause no problems, but sometimes it is excessive and problematic. The tailbone may be flexed too far forward, or extended too far backward.

**Excessive or abrupt forward flexion of the tailbone can cause multiple problems.**

The baseline position of your tailbone is important because that sets the stage for how internal and external structures and forces will interact with your tailbone.

## Flexed Too Far Forward

Often the tailbone position is too far forward. Normally there is supposed to be just a gentle forward sloping where your lower tailbone gradually curves forward into your pelvis.

Anatomy, like life, is a balance of benefits and risks. The benefit of forward curvature of your lower tailbone is that this helps keep your tailbone "tucked in" and "out-of-the-way" when you sit down. This position helps prevent your tailbone from contacting the chair. This minimizes how much body weight or pressure is placed on your tailbone.

However, sometimes the forward curvature (or flexion) is excessive. Often this excessive forward angle of the lower coccyx occurs abruptly at a single coccygeal joint. For example, between the first bone and second bone of the coccyx there may be a very abrupt, 90 degree angle of forward flexion.

Excessive or abrupt forward flexion of the tailbone can cause multiple problems.

The excessive forward flexion of the coccyx can cause the coccyx to obstruct bowel movements. The rectum (a lower part of the large intestine) is located just in front of the tailbone. If the tailbone is flexed too far forward then it makes contact with the back wall of the rectum. The tailbone pushes into the rectum. Sometimes on an

MRI we can see that the forward-flexed coccyx is pushing so far against the rectum that it causes a visible indentation into the rectum.

How can this indentation into the rectum obstruct bowel movements? Well, imagine a garden hose and pushing your thumb forcefully enough to indent the garden hose. If you caused enough indentation, you would obstruct the flow of water through the hose. Water and water pressure would start to back up. Similarly at the rectum, indentation by the coccyx can cause stool to back up. Constipation occurs.

Meanwhile, the water pressure within the hose would be exerting force back onto your thumb. The prolonged, increased pressure in the hose could cause abnormal forces onto the bones and joints within your thumb. Eventually, your thumb would feel sore. Similarly prolonged pressure from the rectum can cause soreness at the tailbone.

Under these circumstances, when you pass stool (have a bowel movement) the force of the stool moving through your rectum can cause sudden pain at the tailbone. Fortunately, only a small percentage of patients with tailbone pain have this kind of exacerbation during bowel movements. But when this occurs it is often because of this indentation phenomenon due to the coccyx being in excessive forward flexion. Most colorectal specialists are unaware that this coccyx problem can cause rectal pain and constipation.

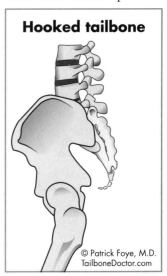

**Hooked tailbone**

© Patrick Foye, M.D.
TailboneDoctor.com

This excessive forward curvature of the tailbone can also create problems when pregnant women go into labor and delivery. During childbirth, the baby passes through the birth canal within the pelvis. If the tailbone is flexed too far forward then it can obstruct the birth canal. The force of the baby's head and shoulders moving through the birth canal can cause the tailbone to dislocate or even fracture. (See Chapter 27: *Pregnancy, Childbirth and Tailbone Pain.*)

## Extended Too Far Backward

Opposite to the problem of a coccyx that is flexed too far forward is the problem of a coccyx that is extended too far backward.

When the tailbone is extended too far backward, it fails to be tucked forward into the pelvis when sitting. The extended tailbone makes earlier and more substantial contact with the chair. This means that sitting causes more weight-bearing pressure onto the tailbone.

This increased force and pressure onto the tailbone during sitting can cause pain and eventually result in arthritis, joint laxity and joint instability.

In addition, the extended tailbone is also less protected from external trauma if you fall onto the tailbone region.

## Summary

The baseline position of the tailbone is important. If the tailbone is flexed too far forward, it can obstruct bowel movements and child-birth. If the tailbone is extended too far backward, it can obstruct sitting. If you have tailbone pain, your physician's evaluation should include a careful physical examination and review of imaging studies to assess the position of your tailbone.

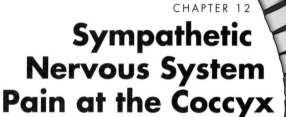

# CHAPTER 12

# Sympathetic Nervous System Pain at the Coccyx

## Linda's Story

Although Linda's tailbone arthritis had previously responded well to local anti-inflammatory steroid injections, the treatments were no longer helping much. She was starting to lose hope, worrying that she may end up having to undergo surgical removal of her tailbone since the injections for her musculoskeletal pain were no longer working very well. In addition, she had developed a type of nerve pain. Linda had excessive sensitivity and irritability of nerve fibers within the sympathetic nervous system. A local anesthetic (lidocaine) nerve block at her ganglion Impar provided her with complete relief.

## What Is the Sympathetic Nervous System?

The nerves throughout your body can be categorized in many different ways. Some nerves are under our voluntary control, such as the nerves that we use to cause our muscles to work, moving our bodies, or lifting something. Some nerves, however, are not under our voluntary or conscious control. These involuntary nerves include the "autonomic nervous system." You can think of the "autonomic" nerves as being "automatic," since they work automatically without you consciously controlling them.

The autonomic nervous system has two main systems (or networks) of nerves: the parasympathetic nervous system and the sympathetic nervous system. In this nerve context, the word "sympathetic" has nothing to do with emotionally feeling sympathy or empathy for our fellow humans.

These autonomic nerve networks function in the background without us needing to think about them or even be aware of them. The parasympathetic and sympathetic nervous systems counteract each other.

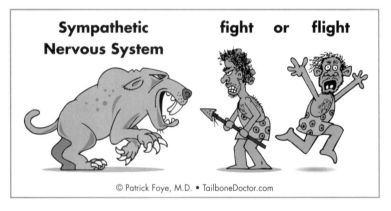

© Patrick Foye, M.D. • TailboneDoctor.com

The parasympathetic nervous system promotes a state of relaxation. Your heart rate and blood pressure are relaxed. Your psychological state is relaxed. Your body can work on background maintenance activities such as digesting food or sleeping.

In contrast to the parasympathetic nervous system, the sympathetic nervous system has the opposite effects. The sympathetic nervous system causes what is commonly known as the "fight or flight" response. This means that if suddenly a lion is approaching you, your body would react and kick into high gear. You would go into a very active state, so that you can either prepare to battle against the lion (fight) or to run away (flight). Heart rate and blood pressure go up. The pupils within your eyes get wider to see more of your surroundings. Resources such as blood flow are diverted from main-tenance activities (such as digesting food within your intestines), and instead are directed to muscles (which will be needed for your fight or flight).

**"Sympathetically Maintained Pain" (SMP) is a pain syndrome due to hyperactivity of the sympathetic nervous system.**

When the threat of injury is over (the lion has been defeated or has gone away), ideally your sympathetic nervous system should quiet back down. Unfortunately, sometimes the sympathetic nervous system stays overactive for a prolonged period. Sometimes this over-activity of the sympathetic nervous system is associated with persistent pain syndromes, such as "Complex Regional Pain Syn-drome" (CRPS) and "Reflex Sympathetic Dystrophy" (RSD).

## What Is "CRPS" and "RSD"?

Complex Regional Pain Syndrome (CRPS) is a condition where an area or region of the body develops severe and often chronic pain. An older term for this was Reflex Sympathetic Dystrophy (RSD). Although CRPS most commonly affects the limbs (such as a foot or hand), it can occur in other regions throughout the body. The full details of this complex condition are beyond the scope of this book. But one hallmark of CPRS is that a patient has pain out of proportion to the stimuli placed upon that body region. For example, even lightly pressing upon the involved body region can be associ-ated with severe pain. In many cases, CRPS is associated with hyper-activity of the sympathetic nervous system.

## What Is "Sympathetically Maintained Pain"?

"Sympathetically Maintained Pain" is a pain syndrome due to hyperactivity of the sympathetic nervous system. The phenomenon is complex and only partly understood. It's like the body region is in a perpetual state of excessive readiness for battle. That body region may be excessively attuned to perceiving external stimuli, such as mild pressure that your body would normally not even notice when you are in a more relaxed state.

Because hyperactivity of the sympathetic nervous system is an underlying cause of Sympathetically Maintained Pain, shutting off the sympathetic nervous system may provide relief of pain. This is accomplished by putting a local anesthetic, such as Lidocaine, onto those sympathetic nerves by performing a local injection. The local anesthetic shuts off the nerve function, so it is called a nerve block. Specifically, in this case the injection is shutting off the sympathetic nerve fibers, so it is called a sympathetic nerve block. If a sympathetic nerve block relieves your pain, this confirms that the sympathetic nervous system had indeed been a cause of your pain syndrome.

## How Is This Relevant to Tailbone Pain?

The sympathetic nervous system travels in a network of nerve pathways throughout the body. Just like a network of trains has hubs or train stations where multiple train lines converge, the nerve network also has hubs. A nerve hub is called a "ganglion." (When there is more than one ganglion, the plural term is ganglia.) The ganglia for the sympathetic nervous system run along the human vertebral spine. From these hubs (ganglia) along the spine, the nerves branch out to travel to other body regions, such as the arms and legs.

Interestingly, the very final or lowest hub (ganglion) of the sympathetic nervous system is located at the front of the upper coccyx. This specific sympathetic nerve hub is called the "ganglion

Impar." Even more interesting and important is that hyperactivity of the ganglion Impar seems to cause sympathetically maintained pain in the tailbone region.

Admittedly, Sympathetically Maintained Pain (SMP) in the tailbone region does not have all of the features associated with CRPS (RSD) in the limbs. For example, CRPS in the hands or feet are often associated with changes in the growth of the fingernails or toenails. Of course there are no such fingernails or toenails that can be involved in the coccyx region. Also, CRPS in the hands or feet are often associated with a difference in skin temperature and skin color when comparing one side to the other (right versus left). Of course, there is no such right versus left comparison possible at the tailbone, since the tailbone is located at the midline of the human body.

But there are two important factors that SMP of the coccyx has in common with SMP within the limbs. First, many patients with coccyx pain suffer from pain that is out of proportion to the external stimuli. Just as many patients with SMP of the hands or feet will feel severe pain from even mild pressure upon their hands or feet, many patients with coccyx pain will feel severe pain from even mild pressure upon the coccyx.

Second, just as many patients with SMP of the hands or feet experience dramatic relief from treatment with a sympathetic nerve block, so too do many patients with coccyx pain experience dramatic relief from a coccygeal sympathetic nerve block (ganglion Impar block). These coccygeal sympathetic nerve blocks are injections that put local anesthetics at the ganglion Impar. This will be discussed in depth in the chapter on treatment using coccyx injections. (See Chapter 24: *Injections for Tailbone Pain*.)

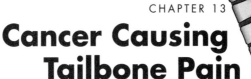

CHAPTER 13

# Cancer Causing Tailbone Pain

### Susan's Story

Susan's local doctor had treated her tailbone pain for more than a year without getting any adequate imaging tests of the painful area. When she flew in for evaluation here at the Tailbone Pain Center, we ordered advanced medical imaging studies. We discovered a bone cancer known as chordoma, which was eating away at her sacrum and coccyx. Unfortunately, this bone cancer often occurs at the coccyx and is often deadly.

**There are multiple cancers that can involve the tailbone region.**

Treatment required extensive surgery to remove her entire coccyx, most of her sacrum, and part of her colon. Surgical removal of Susan's cancer prevented the malignancy from spreading further, thereby saving her life. She continues to be monitored very closely since this particular cancer has a high rate of recurrence.

### Cancer Causing Tailbone Pain

Unfortunately, there are multiple cancers that can involve the tailbone region. For this discussion, I will interchangeably use the terms cancer and malignancy. It is probably best to start by classifying these tailbone malignancies as being either cancers which start within the coccyx itself versus cancers that start someplace else but travel (spread) to the coccyx.

The coccyx is, of course, made of bone and therefore can be a site for bone cancer. Probably the most concerning bone cancer in the sacrococcygeal (sacrum and coccyx) region is chordoma. Chordoma is a "primary" bone cancer, which means that it originates from within bone, rather than originating in other tissue and spreading to the bone. Chordoma is a very aggressive cancer, with aggressive meaning that it can quickly grow, spread, destroy and kill.

There are five main reasons why I worry about chordoma in patients with tailbone pain.

*First*, chordoma has a tendency to occur specifically at the sacrum and coccyx. So chordoma is more likely to be seen in patients with tailbone pain as compared with patients with foot pain or hand pain, for example.

*Second*, chordoma has a high fatality rate, causing death in most of those who have it.

*Third*, the treatment for chordoma is very extensive, including surgical removal of the coccyx and most or all of the sacrum, along with much of the surrounding tissues, such as the rectum. Because this cancer is so aggressive, the treating surgeon must remove a large area of the body in hopes of removing all of the cancer, including removing any cancer cells that may have spread beyond the borders of the sacrum and coccyx.

*Fourth*, even with such extensive surgical treatment, chordoma unfortunately has a high recurrence rate. This means that even if treatment was initially thought to have removed all the cancer, this malignancy may be discovered again within the patient, often a few years later.

*Fifth*, chordoma can fail to show up on typical x-rays. Even in cases where the x-ray images look normal, there can be substantial underlying bone destruction from chordoma.

## Cancers Near the Tailbone Region

There are a variety of cancers originating outside of the coccyx that can cause pain in the coccyx region. These cancers can cause pain in the coccyx region either by the cancer just having a pain referral pattern that includes the coccyx region or by the cancer actually spreading (metastasizing) to the tailbone.

For example, a patient may have rectal cancer. The rectum is the part of the large intestine where stool collects before a bowel movement. It is located just in front of the coccyx. Pain from rectal cancer may be poorly localized (that is, the patient may not be exactly sure where the pain is coming from). But the area of discomfort can include the tailbone region. That patient may feel pain in the tailbone (or tailbone region), but the underlying cause is deeper, within the rectum. Further, the rectal cancer itself may have spread beyond the rectum, invading into the tailbone or sacrum. So the difference is whether just the *pain* is spreading to the tailbone versus whether the *cancer itself* is spreading to the tailbone.

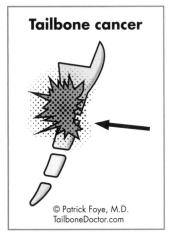

**Tailbone cancer**

© Patrick Foye, M.D.
TailboneDoctor.com

There are similar concerns with other pelvic cancers. In women, common pelvic cancers include malignancies of the cervix, ovaries, and uterus. In men, prostate cancer is very common. For any of these, the cancer may cause pain that refers (travels) to the tailbone region and thus may present with a symptom of tailbone pain. This can happen even if the malignancy has not actually invaded the tailbone. Also, these cancers which start within the cervix, ovaries, uterus, or prostate may actually spread (invade) into the coccyx. Thus, the coccyx area can become associated with the cancer either indirectly (referred pain) or directly (spread of the cancer).

## Symptoms of an Underlying Cancer

Symptoms of an underlying cancer can be categorized as being either generalized or local. Generalized symptoms would include unexplained weight loss, night sweats, lack of energy, and overall feeling unwell.

Local symptoms of an underlying cancer would depend upon the site of the specific cancer. For example, rectal cancer can cause blood in the stool or other changes in bowel movements. A tumor (mass) behind the back of the rectum (such as a retrorectal hamartoma) may create pressure on the rectum, causing the person to feel like he/she needs to have a bowel movement even when there is no stool present. Women with cancer of the cervix may have an abnormal amount of vaginal bleeding or pain with sexual intercourse. Men with prostate cancer may have abnormally frequent or difficult urination.

If you have tailbone pain and any additional generalized or local symptoms, you should inform your treating physician so that appropriate testing can be done.

## Physician Specialists for Cancer Screening

If you are concerned that an underlying cancer may be causing your tailbone pain, see your primary care physician (such as an internal medicine physician or family practice physician).

If you or your physician suspect a specific type of cancer, then see a specialist in that area. For example, people concerned about rectal cancer should see a gastroenterologist. A woman concerned about cancer of her reproductive organs (for example, cancer of the cervix, uterus or ovaries) should see her gynecologist. Similarly, a man concerned about prostate cancer should see a urologist. For tailbone pain patients who have a history of a previous cancer (especially if this was a cancer within the pelvic area) you should ideally follow up with the previous treating physician for that cancer, since he/she will know your prior history and your risk of possible return (recurrence) of the prior cancer.

## Imaging Studies to Show an Underlying Cancer

X-rays are often the first imaging studies done in patients with tailbone pain. However, x-rays are not considered a good test for detecting cancer in patients with tailbone pain. X-rays can completely fail at detecting cancers located within structures other than bones (such as cancers within the rectum, urinary bladder or within the male or female reproductive organs). Meanwhile, although x-rays may detect cancer located within bone, they usually would only be successful in doing so if the cancer had already caused substantial destruction of the bones. For these reasons, x-rays provide only partial reassurance against malignancy in a patient with tailbone pain. To detect cancers, superior tests may include MRIs, CT scans, and nuclear medicine bone scans.

MRI and CT scans in the pelvic region offer images of multiple organ systems. Comparing MRI versus CT scans, there are differences in cost, diagnostic abilities, and radiation exposure. Pelvic MRI may detect cancer within the prostate, uterus, ovaries, rectum, retro-rectal space (behind the rectum), or within the bones of the sacrum and coccyx. Pelvic CT scans may detect similar types of cancers as MRI can. But CT scans are much less expensive, and thus less likely to need insurance pre-authorization. However, MRI may be superior for detecting soft tissue (non-bone) cancers. Also, a significant negative about CT scans is that they deliver radiation to your pelvic organs, which may increase your risk for future cancers. MRI delivers no such potentially harmful radiation.

Regardless of whether you undergo CT scanning or an MRI, the specific way that the test is performed is crucial for the test to be useful in evaluating your tailbone pain. When a CT scan or MRI of the "pelvic" region is ordered, the test is typically done to look mainly at tissues in the front areas of the pelvis (such as the urinary bladder and female reproductive organs). This means that the pelvic imaging often fails to adequately evaluate the back area of the pelvis, such as the tailbone (where my patients are often having their worst pain). Whenever I am ordering MRI or CT imaging of the pelvis for a patient with tailbone pain, I make sure to very explicitly indicate that the specific additional views needed are to include the painful coccyx. This includes midline sagittal thin "slices" on MRI or CT images of the coccyx. (See Chapter 16: *Medical Tests for Tailbone Pain.*)

Nuclear medicine bone scans can also be done to look for cancer that has spread to bone. Again, doing the test properly is crucial. Unfortunately, bone scan images are typically done in a way that has the nuclear medicine material within the urinary bladder obstructing the view of the coccyx and lower sacrum. That obstructed view of the coccyx could make the test useless in evaluating for cancer involvement of the coccyx. This problem can be avoided by using a side view (lateral view) but only if the physician knows to order the test that way. This helps ensure that the radiology technician will perform the test properly.

## Other Tests for Underlying Cancers

Aside from imaging studies, there are other medical tests to look for underlying cancer in patients with tailbone pain. The most basic "test" is a careful evaluation by your physician (such as your primary care physician, gynecologist, urologist, or gastroenterologist). Detailed evaluation of your history, symptoms and physical examination findings may reveal an abnormality that turns out to be malignant.

Further evaluation would depend upon what type of cancer is being considered. For example, if cancer of the urinary bladder is suspected, a urine analysis may be performed or even a cystoscopy (where a video camera is inserted into the bladder, and then a biopsy can be taken of areas that look suspicious).

There are a variety of gynecologic tests to screen for cancers of a woman's reproductive organs. A Pap smear may be done to check for whether a woman has cervical cancer. During the gynecological speculum exam, a biopsy can be done to obtain tissue from any suspicious areas.

To evaluate the lower portions of the gastrointestinal tract (such as the rectum, which is located just in front of the sacrum and coccyx), a medical procedure can be done to look inside the anus, rectum or colon. These tests include:
- anoscopy - looking just inside the anus,
- proctoscopy - looking further, into the rectum,
- sigmoidoscopy - looking further, into the rectum and sigmoid colon, and
- colonoscopy - looking even further, into the entire colon.

## How Are These Underlying Cancers Treated?

The treatment of an underlying cancer depends upon the specific location, the type of cancer, and whether or not it has spread. Treatments can vary from watchful waiting (observation over time), to chemotherapy, to radiation treatment, to surgical excision (removal). This is obviously an over-simplified summary of the cancer treatment options. Consultation with a cancer specialist (oncologist) may be needed.

The most important take-home point is that earlier detection usually results in the cancer being much more treatable, and much less likely to cause more widespread illnesses or even death. For these reasons, I routinely ask my tailbone patients to follow up regularly with their local treating physicians (such as primary care doctors and gynecologists) and to be evaluated by the appropriate specialist if there are significant concerns.

## Free Bonus for You

For your free printable checklist to screen for cancers of the tailbone region, go to: **TailboneDoctor.com/forms**

# CHAPTER 14

# Bone Infection Causing Coccyx Pain

## James's Story

After his heart attack, James's medical complications resulted in weeks of inpatient hospitalization. While there, he developed a bedsore (skin breakdown) over the sacrum and coccyx. Although the overlying skin healed, an underlying pain still persisted months later. He also suffered from an overall feeling of fatigue. Eventually, he came to the Tailbone Pain Center. Our evaluation revealed that the bedsore had caused an underlying bone infection (osteomyelitis) of the coccyx. Even though the overlying skin had healed, the underlying bone infection had persisted. This was subsequently cured with a special regimen of antibiotic treatments.

## How Common Is Bone Infection as a Source of Tailbone Pain?

Infection of the actual bones of the coccyx is not particularly common, but it is crucial to recognize infection if it is indeed present. Out of every hundred patients who I evaluate for tailbone pain, there is probably only one patient

(1 percent) where I end up having a substantial concern about a possible infection of the underlying bone. Still, it is crucial to screen for these uncommon cases, since the treatment for an infection is dramatically different than treatment for other causes of tailbone pain.

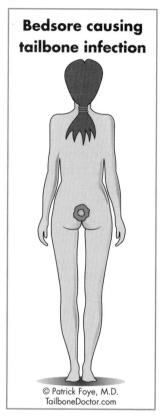

**Bedsore causing tailbone infection**

© Patrick Foye, M.D.
TailboneDoctor.com

## Risk Factors for Bone Infection at the Coccyx

The most common risk factors for a current infection in the coccygeal bones would be a history of previous infection or skin breakdown in the tailbone region. For example, I have seen many patients with a history of bedsores (skin breakdown behind the sacrum and coccyx). Bedsores in the sacrococcygeal region (also called pressure ulcers, or decubitus ulcers) result from someone spending extended time in bed, lying on their back without moving often enough. Sometimes the pressure ulcer is so severe that the skin and underlying soft tissue have entirely eroded away, leaving the underlying sacrococcygeal bones exposed. Exposed bones are at risk for becoming infected. So, in a patient who had a pressure ulcer (with or without any history of local infection at the time of the pressure ulcer), it is worthwhile to consider that the underlying sacral and coccygeal bones may indeed now be harboring an infection.

Similarly, patients who have undergone coccygectomy (surgical amputation of the tailbone) are at risk for bone infection at the surgical site. The remaining bones of the upper coccyx or lower sacrum may become infected during the weeks or months after the surgery. So, the possibility of infection needs to be considered in people who have persistent or worsening pain after coccygectomy. (See Chapter 25: *Coccygectomy: Surgical Removal of the Tailbone*)

Bone infection is called osteomyelitis. Specifically, osteomyelitis is infection within the substance of the bone itself, rather than being an infection in the soft tissue surrounding the bone.

As discussed above, sacrococcygeal bone infection can occur through direct exposure caused by local pressure ulcers or by coccygectomy surgery. However, bone infection can also occur as a result of spread from distant body sites. For example, a patient may have a urinary tract infection, pneumonia (lung infection), or another site of primary infection. Some of the bacteria from the primary infection site may travel through the bloodstream to other body regions, including to the coccyx. Doctors call this hematogenous spread. From the bloodstream, the bacteria can "seed" or settle into these distant body regions, including settling within bone.

**Osteomyelitis is infection within the substance of the bone.**

Thus, since bone infection can occur either by direct extension into the bone or by blood-borne spread from distant sites, any significant previous infection in the body can potentially be considered a risk factor for coccygeal bone infection as the cause of tailbone pain.

## Symptoms of Tailbone Infection

Underlying bone infection can cause symptoms such as unexplained fevers, chills, night sweats, and weight loss. In addition to those generalized symptoms throughout the body, local symptoms at the site of a bone infection could include pain in that area. Other local symptoms may include redness, swelling, or warmth of the overlying skin. Note that none of these symptoms are guaranteed to occur with every bone infection case, so the absence of one or more of these does not guarantee that there is no bone infection present.

## Bone Infection Despite Antibiotics

Unfortunately, a bone infection can often continue despite a typical treatment with antibiotics. When you have an infection of your urinary bladder (urinary tract infection), lung (pneumonia), nasal sinuses (bacterial sinusitis), skin (cellulitis), or other body regions, you are often treated with 5 to 10 days of antibiotics by mouth. That short duration of antibiotics may be perfectly adequate to treat your urinary, lung or skin infection.

However, a bacterial infection that is deep within your bone can often survive beyond the 5 to 10 days of antibiotic treatment. So, short-term antibiotics may resolve your symptoms at your nasal sinuses, lungs, urinary bladder, or skin. You and your doctor may then think that you are completely cured, but if there is still some bacterial infection persisting within your bone then a problem is still brewing. After the antibiotics have stopped, your bone infection continues smoldering in the background.

After a while, you may once again start having fevers, chills, night sweats, or similar generalized symptoms. You and your physician may be unaware of the source or site of the current infection. Sometimes another 5 to 10 days of antibiotics are given, which again just quiets things down temporarily but fails to completely remove the infection from deep within your bone. Sometimes these cycles of short-term antibiotics are repeated multiple times, with each time giving you and your physician a false sense of victory since your generalized fever, chills, and night sweats get better temporarily. As we will discuss later in this chapter, it is crucial to diagnose the underlying bone infection and treat it with a much longer and better course of antibiotics.

## Diagnosing Osteomyelitis (Bone Infection)

The diagnosis of osteomyelitis is based upon your medical history, symptoms, physical exam findings, and test results.

We have already discussed the symptoms (including both generalized symptom such as unexplained fevers, chills, night sweats, weight loss, and localized symptoms such as focal pain). Physical exam findings may include pain or tenderness when pressing on the area, as well as redness, swelling or warmth of the overlying skin.

Diagnostic tests for osteomyelitis include bloodwork, imaging studies, and sometimes a bone biopsy. The bloodwork usually includes a CBC (complete blood count), specifically looking for signs of infection such as an abnormally high number of white blood cells (WBCs). Further blood tests can look for overall inflammation, such as elevation of the Erythrocyte Sedimentation Rate (ESR) and C-reactive proteins (CRP). So, elevation in WBCs, ESR, and CRP are all suggestive for underlying inflammation, as occurs with an infection. However, those test results do not specifically indicate the part of the body where the inflammation or infection is occurring.

Imaging studies are helpful since they may reveal abnormalities at the specific site of bone infection. Plain x-rays may fail to detect a bone infection until substantial bone destruction has already taken place. CT scans and MRIs are much better than x-rays at detecting osteomyelitis.

Another imaging study that can be done to check for osteo-myelitis is a triple phase (three phase) bone scan. This type of bone scan is also called skeletal skintigraphy and is very different than the bone "density" scan done to check for osteoporosis. Triple phase bone scans are typically done in the nuclear medicine section of a radiology department since they involve injecting radioactive tracer material into the bloodstream. Images taken over the course of multiple hours assess for "hot-spots" showing areas of bone destruction. To assess for osteomyelitis specifically at the tailbone or lower sacrum, it is crucial that the bone scan include all three phases and that it also include views looking at the pelvis from the side (lateral) perspective.

CT scans, MRIs, and bone scans are discussed in further detail in the chapter on diagnostic imaging. (See Chapter 16: *Medical Tests for Tailbone Pain*.)

## Labeled White Blood Cell (WBC) Scan

White blood cells (WBCs) are part of the immune system, which fights infections. These cells travel through the bloodstream to a site of infection. White blood cell function is assessed by the white blood cell labeled scan (also called labeled leukocyte imaging). Blood is drawn from a patient's vein (usually in the arm) and the cells are taken from this blood sample. The blood cells are then labeled, or tagged, by having a detectable radioactive chemical (such as indium, gallium or technetium) attached to them.

These labeled white blood cells are then injected back into the bloodstream. Since these cells naturally travel to the site of infection, they should pool (collect) at any body region where infection is actively occurring. Images done hours later can then detect the tracer material, showing whether the labeled blood cells have collected at the coccyx (which would suggest local infection at that site).

The white blood cell labeled scan is not commonly performed. It does have some limitations, such as false positive results since it may be difficult to distinguish infection from other types of inflammation. (These cells may collect at any site of inflammation, not only sites of infection.) However, the results can be an important "piece of the puzzle" in cases where there is a significant concern regarding infection in the coccyx region, especially when other tests (such as bloodwork and MRIs) have failed to conclusively answer whether infection is present or not.

## Treating Bone Infections

As stated above, bone infections require a longer duration of antibiotic treatment than is needed for most other infections. The typical 5 to 10 days of antibiotics taken by mouth may work perfectly fine for most infections of the skin, urinary bladder and other organs. But that antibiotic approach would be woefully inadequate for treating a bone infection.

So, to treat infection deep within the bone, antibiotics are often given for a full six weeks. This longer duration helps to ensure that any "smoldering" infection (lingering bacteria) within bone is more thoroughly killed. The goal, of course, is to kill not just 99 percent of the bacteria; the goal is to kill them all.

Bone infections may require the antibiotics to be given intravenously rather than by mouth. This means that a needle needs to be inserted into a blood vessel (a vein or artery) and the antibiotic is then delivered directly into the bloodstream.

The antibiotics for treating bone infection may combine the first week or two of antibiotics being given intravenously (perhaps while hospitalized), followed by the remainder of the six weeks of antibiotics being given by mouth at home. If the entire six weeks need to be given directly into the bloodstream (intravenously—IV), the patient can sometimes receive this IV at home after placement of a special type of access to their bloodstream (such as a PIC line, which is an abbreviation for a peripherally inserted central line). This type of access to the bloodstream can allow many patients to have their six weeks of antibiotics administered at home perhaps by a visiting nurse coming to the home each day, instead of needing to remain in the hospital.

Another difference in the treatment of bone infection may be the specific antibiotic that is chosen. The antibiotic given should be one that is effective at treating the specific bacteria that is causing the infection. In many body regions, it's relatively easy to find out what antibiotic will work against the infection. For example, with a urinary tract (bladder) infection, the patient can urinate into a cup and subsequent testing can reveal what bacteria are present and what antibiotics will work against those bacteria. Similarly, for pneumonia the patient can cough up a sputum sample which is tested to reveal the bacteria and its antibiotic sensitivity. Skin infection (cellulitis) can simply be "swabbed" at the infected skin site to obtain the necessary sample for testing.

But infection within bone creates significant difficulties in obtaining a sample of the bacteria. Obtaining a sample of infected bony material requires drilling or cutting into the bone and removing a small piece of the bone (a bone biopsy). Obviously this is much more invasive and destructive than the simple ways that bacterial samples are obtained for infections of the urinary bladder, lungs or skin.

## Underlying Medical Conditions That Put You at Risk for Bone Infection

Medical risks for bone infection include local breakdown of the skin over the sacrum or coccyx, which occurs with bedsores (pressure ulcers) and with surgical removal of the tailbone. Also, distant infections from other body regions can cause bacteria to spread through the bloodstream and settle into a bony area where a new infection site takes hold.

Further, some patients have underlying medical illnesses that predispose them to infections. For example, patients with cancer, HIV (human immunodeficiency virus) or AIDS (acquired immunodeficiency syndrome) often have immune system impairments that raise the risk of infection taking hold.

## Tuberculosis (TB) Infection Causing Tailbone Pain

Tuberculosis (commonly referred to as TB) is a bacterial infection that typically involves the lungs. TB is more common in parts of Asia and Africa, as well as within certain populations in the United States, such as among prisoners.

Although TB typically starts as a lung infection, it can spread to the bones of the vertebral spine (called Pott's disease). The vertebral bones most commonly infected are those of the thoracic spine, which are the spinal bones closest to the lungs. However, TB can instead spread to the spinal bones of the sacrum and coccyx.

Suspect possible TB infection of the coccyx region if you have a history of the following:
- pulmonary (lung) TB infection,
- a positive skin test (PPD test) for TB,
- travel to areas where TB is common, or
- an underlying condition that causes decreased ability of the immune system to fight infections.

The tuberculosis bacteria are often resistant to many antibiotics and thus treatment often requires giving multiple antibiotics to the patient at the same time.

## Medical Specialists for Bone Infection

Usually you should start by seeing your primary care physician for evaluation of infection as a possible cause of your pain. If you have HIV infection, AIDS, or cancer, then you should continue to follow closely with the physicians already treating you for those conditions.

It may be worthwhile to consult a physician specializing in infectious diseases (ID). Also, an orthopedic surgeon may be required if a bone biopsy is needed. For example, a bone sample can be obtained and cultured to see if it really is infected and to see what antibiotics the infection should be treated with.

## Infections Other Than Bone

Because tissues such as skin, muscles, and tendons are much "softer" than bone, infections in those softer tissues are often referred to as "soft tissue infections." Infection of the skin (cellulitis) usually results in the skin being red in color and warm to the touch. A skin infection may spread widely throughout the skin or may remain in a more localized lump. For example, a carbuncle is a focal skin infection that forms a lump and may contain pus.

Another example of a lump in the skin is a pilonidal cyst. A pilonidal cyst is a sac (or pocket) of hair and debris in the skin in the tailbone region. This can become infected, forming into a pilonidal abscess. Treatment may include antibiotics and surgical removal of the cyst.

Since the coccyx is very close to the anus, anal infections (such as a perianal abscess) can also cause pain in the coccyx region. Sometimes, internal evaluation of the anus and rectum may be necessary, including consultation with a gastroenterologist.

## Free Bonus for You

For your free printable checklist screening for infections of the tailbone region, go to: **TailboneDoctor.com/forms**

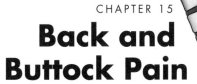

# CHAPTER 15

# Back and Buttock Pain

## Mary's Story

To minimize her tailbone pain, Mary often sat leaning sideways onto just one buttock, or sat leaning forward. But these abnormal sitting positions caused abnormal mechanical stresses on other parts of her body. After many months of this, she started having additional pain up at her belt line area (lower back) as well as at her buttocks and down into her legs. When Mary came to our Tailbone Pain Center, we diagnosed lumbar facet joint pain, piriformis muscle pain, and sciatica. She felt that her tailbone pain was definitely the worst of these symptoms. We felt that the other problems were mostly due to the abnormal sitting postures. Treating and resolving her tailbone pain allowed Mary to sit normally again. Over the next several weeks, all of her other symptoms disappeared.

## Pain at Areas Other Than the Tailbone

There are multiple reasons why a book on tailbone pain needs to cover other sources of pain in the low back and buttock region. For starters, many patients come to me with the unfortunate experience of having had their tailbone problems incorrectly labeled as other types of lower back pain syndromes. My hope is that this chapter will help you to distinguish between these different sources of pain and help you to be on guard against having the source of your pain incorrectly diagnosed or incorrectly labeled.

Many people have a poor sense of "body awareness" for the physical structures within their lower back and pelvic region. If I asked you to touch your right pinky finger and right biceps muscle, you would probably know

**Abnormal sitting positions (due to tailbone pain) can cause pain in the low back, buttocks and legs.**

exactly where those are, without hesitation. But if I asked you to touch over your right lower lumbar zygapophyseal joints, ischial bursa, or piriformis muscle, you may be uncertain about these. By empowering you to understand all of these (and more), this chapter seeks to decrease your chances of being incorrectly diagnosed (mis-diagnosed) with medical conditions at those sites. Part of confidently determining that your pain is coming from the tailbone requires making sure that your pain is *not* coming from other nearby sites.

Further, patients with tailbone pain often *do* have additional pain at some of these other nearby sites. Often this comes from weeks, months or years of trying to decrease tailbone pain by sitting in abnormal body positions. Many patients with tailbone pain try to ease their tailbone pain by sitting leaning forward or sitting lean-ing toward one side or the other (onto the right or left buttock). Those sitting positions can help decrease the severity of tailbone pain while sitting.

But there is a cost. Prolonged time in abnormal body positions can cause musculoskeletal pain in other nearby body regions. Abnormal sitting positions due to tailbone pain can cause pain in the low back, buttocks and legs. Thus, your pain may no longer be limited to only your tailbone. Treatment may require first treating the underlying tailbone pain, and then additionally treating any pain that lingers at the other involved areas. This is important since treatment of the secondary problems without treating the underlying tailbone problem may result in minimal or merely temporary relief at those sites (since the tailbone pain continues to cause the abnormal sitting postures).

Although this chapter will cover many of the most common causes of pain in the general lower back and buttock region, there's no way that a single chapter could cover them all or cover them in depth. This chapter seeks to give enough of an overview, though, to point you in the right direction.

## Low Back Pain

The term "low back pain" (or lumbago) refers to pain or discomfort essentially anywhere in the lower back (lumbar) region. A huge problem with the general phrase "low back pain" is that it fails to specify the actual specific site or cause of the pain. Patients use the term "low back pain" because they do not know the underlying specific anatomy of exactly where the pain is coming from. Low back pain is an umbrella phrase that includes many specific sites that can cause pain.

Using this as a catch-all phrase is common not only among patients but also among many physicians. But if the physician fails to try to make a more specific diagnosis then this nonspecific approach can hinder you from receiving appropriate testing and treatment. Sometimes using the nonspecific label is called the "black box" approach. It implies that the physician is unaware of the various specific components and instead the entire body region is like one big black box. The black box approach is problematic. The more specific we can be at finding the source (or sources) of a

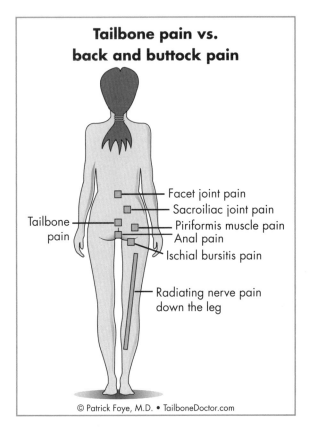

Tailbone pain vs. back and buttock pain

Facet joint pain
Sacroiliac joint pain
Piriformis muscle pain
Anal pain
Ischial bursitis pain
Tailbone pain
Radiating nerve pain down the leg

© Patrick Foye, M.D. • TailboneDoctor.com

person's pain, the more specific we can be with appropriate testing and treatment. So, while we often continue to use the phrase low back pain as a shorthand, general term, the goal should still be to find the specific source of pain.

## Where Is the Lumbar Region?

The first (or uppermost) lumbar vertebral bone (L1, for lumbar-one) is the highest spinal (vertebral) bone in the region that does *not* have a rib attached. (The vertebral bones that do have ribs attached are called the "thoracic" spine.) The lumbar spine typically includes five lumbar vertebral bones. These vertebral bones are stacked one on top of the other. In between the stacked vertebral bodies are intervertebral discs, which act as shock absorbers when force or load is placed upon the spine. The lowest part of the lumbar spine is the fifth lumbar vertebral bone (L5). Below the lumbar spine is the sacral spine (or sacrum), which is typically five vertebral bones fused together (S1 through S5).

Most patients with low back pain experience their pain around the area of L4, L5, and S1. For reference, this is approximately where the belt line or waistband of your pants crosses the small of your back. Note that this area is very different from the tailbone, which is much lower, below the sacrum.

## Lumbar Herniated Disc (Slipped Disc)

Your discs act as shock absorbers in between your vertebral bones. Sometimes the walls, or lining, of the discs become worn out, either gradually or suddenly. The disc can bulge outward, into the spinal canal. Some of the gel-like material from inside the disc can leak or ooze through a tear in the disc wall, causing local irritation and inflammation. The disc wall and disc material has then extended, or herniated, beyond its normal location. Common terms for this include bulging disc, herniated disc, or slipped disc. The pressure and inflammation can cause low back pain around that disc level. The most common levels for lumbar disc herniations are L4-L5 and L5-S1, which are approximately at the belt line. This pain is often worse with activities like lifting, carrying, bending forward while standing, or sometimes with prolonged sitting.

The typical medical test used to diagnose a disc herniation is an MRI. However, an MRI often shows disc bulges and herniations that are not causing the patient any symptoms whatsoever. Many patients who come to see me for tailbone pain report that their previous physician had them undergo a lumbar MRI (which typically does not even include imaging of the tailbone) only to have the lumbar MRI reveal an "abnormality" such as a lumbar disc bulge or herniation. Many of these patients were then unfortunately told that the lumbar disc was the source of their pain, when in reality the lumbar disc was just an "incidental" MRI finding. Unfortunately, many of these patients have even been subjected to lumbar spine injections and even lumbar spine surgery, without any relief of their tailbone pain.

## Lumbar Radiculopathy

In medicine, "radic" means "root," for example, referring to the nerve root as it leaves the spine. The suffix "-pathy" refers to an abnormal condition. Lumbar radiculopathy, then, is an abnormal condition of a nerve root that is leaving the lumbar spine. Since the lumbar spinal nerves travel down into the legs, a right lumbar radiculopathy usually causes pain, numbness, or weakness down into the right leg. People commonly refer to this as having "sciatica," or a "pinched nerve" in their lower back. Common causes for radiculopathy include disc herniations causing pressure or inflammation of the nerve root.

These symptoms can usually be distinguished very clearly from tailbone pain in three ways.

• First, the lumbar discs and nerves are much higher in the body than the tailbone, with the lumbar region being located around the waistband or belt line region while the coccyx is much lower, closer to the anus.

• Second, lumbar radiculopathy will often cause neurologic symptoms (such as pain, numbness, or weakness) traveling down one leg, beyond the knee. By comparison, tailbone pain typically stays midline and would not be expected to cause symptoms traveling beyond the pelvic region.

• Third, pressing externally on the back of the tailbone usually worsens tailbone pain, whereas pressing there would not have any effect on lumbar radiculopathy.

## Lumbar Facet Joint Pain

The lumbar facet joints are also called zygapophyseal joints (also spelled as zygoapophyseal or zygapophysial). These are small, bilateral (right and left) joints between one level of the spine and the next level above or below it. These joints can experience arthritis from wear and tear over the decades. Patients with lumbar facet joint pain typically report stiffness or soreness at about the belt line in the small of the back. The pain is usually worse when leaning backward (lumbar extension). This pain usually stays in that region, without traveling down the leg.

## Sacroiliac Joint (SI Joint) Pain

The sacrum includes five sacral vertebral bones, fused together at the back of the pelvis. The sacrum is below the lumbar spine but above the coccyx. When you look from behind, the sacrum looks like an upside down triangle, more narrow at the bottom and wider across the top. On each side (right and left) the sacrum meets the iliac bone, forming the right and left sacroiliac joints.

Patients with sacroiliac joint arthritis or other painful conditions will typically report pain in the upper buttock on that side. The pain may travel (radiate) to the front of the groin on that same side. Although these sacroiliac joints are lower than the lumbar spine, they are still significantly higher than the tailbone. A careful history and physical examination can often reveal where the pain is coming from. Sometimes, a diagnostic injection (test injection) of local anesthetic (numbing medication) into the SI joint is done to confirm the SI joint as a source of pain.

## Piriformis Muscle Pain

The piriformis muscle starts in front of the sacroiliac joint and from there it angles diagonally toward the lower and outer part of the buttock, heading over to its insertion site at the outer hip region. Muscle spasm at the piriformis typically causes buttock pain on one side or the other. Although the piriformis is somewhat closer to the coccyx than lumbar or sacroiliac joint problems are, the piriformis location is typically far enough from midline to be easily distinguished from tailbone pain with a physician's (or physical therapist's) careful physical exam.

## Piriformis Syndrome

In addition to the piriformis muscle pain discussed above, sometimes muscle spasm at the piriformis can cause irritation of the sciatic nerve. This is called piriformis syndrome. The sciatic nerve is the largest nerve innervating the leg, and as it travels in the buttock region it is just below the piriformis muscle. In some cases, the sciatic nerve actually travels *through* the piriformis muscle, where it can be compressed and irritated by a piriformis muscle spasm. Since the sciatic nerve then travels down the leg, patients will often report buttock pain that travels down that same leg. In some ways the symptoms are similar to those of lumbar radiculopathy (which also causes nerve pain that travels down into the leg). But a careful physician's physical examination can usually distinguish lumbar radiculopathy from piriformis syndrome.

## Sacral Tarlov Cysts

The medical term "cyst" refers to a bag, or sack, of fluid. Within the sacrum, the cerebrospinal fluid can bulge outward from its normal location in the spinal canal, creating a Tarlov cyst. These

Tarlov cysts are often detected by MRI, and are usually considered "incidental" MRI findings (that is, they are usually *not* felt to be a cause of any symptoms). Some physicians may believe dogmatically that sacral Tarlov cysts can *never* cause patients any symptoms. It is more accurate to say that a sacral Tarlov cyst *usually* does not cause symptoms, but occasionally may. Regardless, a sacral Tarlov cyst is higher up than the tailbone and typically would not be expected to cause tailbone pain.

## Pilonidal Cysts

Unlike the Tarlov cyst located within the sacral bone, a pilonidal cyst is located more superficially, as a lump within the skin at the tailbone region. A pilonidal cyst is a sack that contains hair (pilonidal literally means "a nest of hair"). The cyst may become swollen and inflamed. Some symptoms of pilonidal cysts overlap with those of tailbone diagnoses, since patients have pain in the coccyx region that is worse with sitting.

A pilonidal cyst may form a tunnel (called a fistula) through the skin, oozing a fluid that irritates the overlying skin. The cyst or fistula can become infected, forming into a pilonidal abscess. Foul-smelling pus may drain from the abscess. Treatment may require antibiotics and surgical removal of the cyst.

## Pudendal Neuralgia

The pudendal nerve provides innervation (nerve supply) for multiple pelvic areas, including around the anus, the perineum (the area in front of the anus but behind the genitalia), and much of the male and female genitals (including the external genitalia such as the female vulva or the male scrotum and penis). If there is compression or irritation of the pudendal nerve, this can cause nerve pain (neuralgia) in the areas innervated by that nerve. Pudendal neuralgia (also called pudendal neuropathy) can occur in Alcock's canal, where the nerve is particularly susceptible to entrapment or compression. Pressure on this nerve while sitting on a bicycle seat is one risk factor. Patients with pudendal neuralgia often have pain while sitting. Unlike typical coccyx pain, which tends to stay back at the coccyx and at the midline, pudendal neuralgia pain tends to be located farther forward (in the genital region) and is often non-symmetric (mainly affecting either the left side or the right side of the body).

## Pelvic Floor Pain

Pelvic floor pain is an umbrella term that includes a variety of causes of pain in the lower pelvic region. The pelvic floor is like a hammock or sling which holds up the pelvic contents (such as the urinary bladder, uterus, and rectum). The pelvic floor is composed of muscles, tendons and ligaments. Most people are not conscious of the muscles and tendons within their pelvic floor. These structures typically function quietly in the background, usually without causing any problems. However, in some individuals the pelvic floor structures can become painful and dramatically decrease the person's quality of life.

The full spectrum of pelvic floor abnormalities is beyond the scope of this book. There are entire books and courses dedicated just to the pelvic floor. In general, muscles, tendons and ligaments in the pelvic floor can experience painful muscle spasm, structural tears (of these muscles, tendons or ligaments), and various chronic pain syndromes. Just as these types of structures can experience injuries and pain in other body regions, this can also occur in the pelvic floor region. Sometimes there is a specific, known, traumatic event that starts the problems. In other cases, the underlying cause may be more gradual wear and tear from decades of these structures working to hold up the pelvic contents.

Most people have a poor body awareness of their own pelvic anatomy, so patients with pelvic floor pain may be unable to automatically understand or pinpoint what specific structure is causing the pain. The area of pain can span (from back to front) the coccyx, the area around the anus, the perineum (the area from the anus to the base of the external genitalia), and the genital region.

Sometimes the pelvic floor muscles may be so weak that they sag downward, as gravity pulls the pelvic contents down toward the ground. This weakness and sagging can cause pelvic floor "prolapse," where the lower part of the urinary bladder, vagina, uterus, or rectum start to droop or extend (prolapse) lower than the usual confines of the pelvic floor. This can cause pain and also difficulties with urination, sexual intercourse or bowel movements.

Pelvic floor abnormalities are most commonly evaluated by obstetricians/gynecologists (some of whom specifically specialize in pelvic pain syndromes) and specially trained physical therapists. Although most physical therapists do not specialize in the pelvic floor area, there are a growing number who do so and they can be well worth finding. There are also a few PM&R (physical medicine and rehabilitation) or other pain management physicians who specialize in this area. Evaluation and treatment often involves internal examination, meaning that the physician or physical therapist will use a gloved hand to insert a few fingers inside the vagina or rectum to identify the specific site of pain and work on muscle relaxation and muscle re-education.

## Ischial Bursitis

The right and left ischial bones are large, major bones of your pelvis. When you are sitting, much of your body weight is pressing down through your right and left ischial bones (at the right and left lower buttocks). The three points of bony contact with the chair are described as being like a "tripod" composed of the right and left ischial bones, along with the coccyx in the midline. When you are suffering from coccyx pain, you may sit leaning to the right or left in order to take some of the sitting pressure off of your coccyx. But this results in additional pressure onto whichever ischial bone you are leaning toward. Prolonged or recurrent pressure onto either or both lower ischial bones can cause inflammation of a bursa (which is like a small bag filled with fluid). This can result in a painful condition called ischial bursitis. Ischial bursitis generally presents with pain in your lower buttock on the right, left or both sides. The pain is usually worse when sitting leaning toward the involved side. The diagnosis can usually be made based upon your symptoms and physical exam findings.

## Treating the Tailbone to Help Other Areas

Often, tailbone pain is the primary cause of the abnormal sitting posture. Then, the abnormal sitting posture results in pain within the lower back (lumbar area), buttocks or legs. So, treating and resolving the tailbone pain can subsequently result in relief in the lower back, buttock and leg pain. However, if symptoms in those body regions persist, they may require medical treatment beyond just treating the tailbone.

### Free Bonus for You
For your free printable pain diagram, where you can document your back, buttock, and tailbone pain, go to: **Tailbone Doctor.com/forms**

# CHAPTER 16

# Medical Tests for Tailbone Pain

## Karen's Story

Karen was diligent in seeing multiple doctors and going for multiple tests for her tailbone pain. She was repeatedly told that her test results were normal and that they failed to show any explanation for her symptoms. Frustrated, she flew in for evaluation at our Tailbone Pain Center. Our review of her previous tests revealed that all of the x-rays, MRIs and CT scans had focused on the *lumbar* spine, without *any* imaging studies that actually included her painful tailbone.

Karen was shocked that so many tests had been done of the *wrong* body region! Next, dedicated medical imaging specifically showing the tailbone clearly revealed the coccyx abnormality that was causing her pain. Standard x-rays showed normal alignment of her coccyx while she was standing, but x-rays done while seated showed abnormal, excessive joint move-ment. She had an unstable joint at her tailbone, confirming a diagnosis of coccygeal dynamic instability. A coccyx MRI revealed no evidence of cancer but did show inflammation at her unstable coccyx joint. Now that Karen finally had undergone the correct tests to diagnose her condition, she could now move forward with considering personalized treatment options.

## Medical Tests for Tailbone Pain

Beyond carefully listening to the patient's history (symptoms) and performing a thorough physical examination, there are a variety of medical tests that can be done in the evaluation of tailbone pain. These tests can include imaging studies such as x-rays, MRI, CT scans and other studies. Less commonly, bloodwork may be ordered. All of these areas will be covered in further depth in this chapter.

## Standard X-rays (Radiographs) of the Coccyx

Routine x-rays of the coccyx typically include a view from the front (medically called an anterior-posterior, or AP, view) and a view from the side (a lateral view). Unfortunately, a standard AP (frontal) view of the pelvis results in the image of the pubic bones (at the front of the pelvis, just above the genital region) blocking (obstructing) the images of the coccyx (at the back of the pelvis). This would be similar to a photograph where a shadow or obstruction blocks the view of the area of interest for the photo. That standard pelvic AP (frontal) view would be adequate for showing the sacrum but totally useless for showing the tailbone. To optimally image the coccyx from the front, the radiology technician needs to tilt the x-ray source so that it comes in from somewhat higher, above the pubic bones (at the front of the pelvis). This tilt results in an image where the pubic bones are no longer blocking the view of the coccyx.

> **If you suffer from tailbone pain but have not yet undergone coccyx x-rays *while you are sitting,* then your diagnostic workup is *not* complete.**

Aside from the tilt issue, a second problem with these frontal view x-rays is that the view of the tailbone can be clouded by stool within the rectum (which is just in front of the coccyx). Air and stool within the rectum is normal, but can make it difficult to see details of the tailbone on frontal view x-rays. The primary solution to this is the second standard view of the tailbone, which is the lateral view (the side view).

There are many benefits to the side view (lateral view) of the coccyx. First, this side view is not obstructed by stool within the rectum or by the pubic bones. Second, this view is ideal for looking at the individual joint spaces between the coccygeal bones. We can see if those joint spaces are fused or not, whether the joint spaces are larger (taller) than normal (which may suggest excessive joint laxity), and whether there is any abnormality in the alignment of the coccygeal bones as they are stacked one on top of the other. Additionally, if a patient has a bone spur extending backward from the lowest tip of his/her coccyx, this, too, is best seen from a side view.

So, the side view is extremely helpful for assessing coccygeal joint fusion, joint space size, bony alignment, and bone spurs.

Unfortunately, there are some challenges with obtaining these side view x-rays. The coccygeal bones are very small in comparison to the other bones in this region, which can cause technical difficulties with seeing the coccygeal bones properly. By comparison, the sacrum, iliac bones, femurs (thigh bones), and lower lumbar vertebral bodies are all many times bigger than a typical coccygeal bone. Taking a lateral view x-ray that includes all of these larger bones can result in the image being optimized to see those larger bones. When this occurs, the small coccygeal bones can appear hazy or washed out. I compare this to taking a photograph of your pinky fingernail in front of a window on a bright, sunny day. The details of the fingernail would be lost or washed out. The solution would be to zoom in on only the fingernail, thereby blocking out most of the bright window and thus limiting how much washout would occur.

The solution for tailbone x-rays is similar. A "coned-down" view is done by attaching a narrow column to the source of the x-rays. This looks somewhat like attaching a long zoom lens to the front of a camera. This coned-down view has many important benefits.

- First, there is less x-ray radiation delivered to body regions that you were not interested in imaging anyway. (Why cause more x-ray radiation than is needed?)

- Second, the coned-down view creates less image "washout" at the tailbone, since the image will be optimized for the bones that are within the image, which is now just mainly the coccyx.

- Third, the coned-down x-ray beams are no longer being delivered to the larger bones of the lumbar spine, pelvis and hips, which means that they will no longer ricochet (scatter or bounce off) from those larger bones. This is important since the ricochet, or scatter, from the larger bones onto the coccyx causes the coccyx image to become hazy.

So, a coned-down image means fewer x-ray beams are delivered to bones *other* than the coccyx, which means there will be less scatter from those other bones. Less scatter means you will have a clearer image of the area you are focusing on, which is the coccyx.

Yet another problem with standard coccyx x-rays is that they are done while the patient is either standing up or lying down. This is a problem because many patients with tailbone pain have little or no pain while they are standing up or lying down. Your tailbone pain is probably at its worst while you are sitting and especially while you are sitting leaning partway backward. So, the typical x-rays done while standing or lying down are not being done in a position that is causing your pain. The solution is to perform dynamic (sitting versus standing) x-rays of the coccyx.

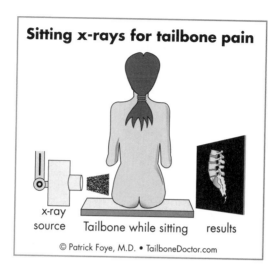

**Sitting x-rays for tailbone pain**

x-ray source    Tailbone while sitting    results

© Patrick Foye, M.D. • TailboneDoctor.com

## Dynamic (Sitting versus Standing) X-rays of the Coccyx

As noted above, most patients with tailbone pain have their worst symptoms while they are sitting and especially while sitting and leaning slightly backward. This is because that position increases the amount of your body weight that is pressing down onto your tailbone.

Decades ago, a physician named Dr. Maigne noticed that patients with coccyx pain often had coccyx x-rays that looked normal while the patients were standing. Dr. Maigne came up with the brilliant idea to do the lateral view coccyx x-ray while a patient was sitting and leaning partly backward. The idea was that these seated x-rays would show the position of the coccygeal bones while the patients were in their most painful position. He quickly discovered that many patients with coccyx x-rays that looked normal while standing were blatantly abnormal while sitting.

Next, Dr. Maigne did research on how much coccygeal movement was normal. He compared the sitting versus standing x-rays in people who had no history of any tailbone pain or tailbone injuries. He found that when going from standing to sitting a small amount of coccygeal movement was normal, and he established cut-offs for how much movement was normal versus abnormal. For example, when people sit the coccyx normally can flex up to 20 degrees. Also, sitting can cause the alignment of one coccygeal bone stacked on top of the other to shift such that there is movement in the amount of overhang (listhesis) by up to 25 percent of the coccygeal vertebral body.

Excessive movement of the coccygeal bones while sitting means that there is an unstable joint within the tailbone. This "dynamic instability" is perhaps the most common cause of tailbone pain. This common diagnosis is usually "missed" (not recognized) because doctors and radiology technicians remain largely unaware of dynamic (sitting versus standing) coccyx x-rays.

Every week in my practice, new patients with tailbone pain come to me saying that their standard x-rays showed a normal coccyx but that no sitting x-rays had yet been done. Often these patients have been told that there is no explanation for their pain. Some have been told that the pain must all just be "in their head" (a figment of their imagination). Sometimes the patients have tried to get their local radiology center to perform the seated coccyx x-rays, only to be incorrectly told that there is no such thing. Very commonly, when we do the sitting versus standing x-rays we discover abnormal, excessive movement at one or more joints within the tailbone, perfectly matching where the patient is having his/her tenderness and pain.

I consider Dr. Maigne's contribution of sitting versus standing coccyx x-rays to be probably the most helpful advancement in the evaluation of tailbone pain in the past half century. If you suffer from tailbone pain but have not yet undergone coccyx x-rays *while you are sitting*, then your diagnostic workup is *not* complete.

## Difficulties with Obtaining Sitting versus Standing Coccyx X-rays

As noted above, a primary difficulty is that many physicians and radiology centers remain completely unaware that seated coccyx x-rays can be performed. They are probably wonderful, caring and experienced healthcare professionals in a million other ways, but they simply lack the knowledge or experience in evaluating tailbone pain. When patients bring them information about seated coccyx x-rays, some clinicians may be willing to try performing these, but with a lack of experience the results are often suboptimal. Some medical professionals become resistant to even trying to perform the test, refusing to accept the information the patient is providing.

Beyond the problems with acceptance by healthcare professionals, there are also some technical challenges in properly performing seated coccyx x-rays. The x-rays are done from a side view (lateral view) of the patient, and the radiology technician must estimate where your coccyx is located to make sure that it is included in the images obtained.

Another technical challenge is that the chair or table needs to be a firm surface (such as wood or hard plastic) because sitting on a cushion may fail to place adequate direct pressure on the tailbone. The chair or table creates technical difficulties for the images since such a dense material is often radio-opaque, meaning that it blocks the x-ray images from getting through. This can make it difficult to deliver just the right amount of x-rays to see the tailbone clearly.

Yet another technical challenge is that other larger bones in the area of the low back, pelvis and upper thigh regions can scatter, or ricochet, x-ray beams causing the image to be hazy. This problem can be minimized by delivering the x-ray beams through a narrow cylinder, creating a coned-down view focusing just on the coccyx area.

With experience and training, proper sit-stand x-rays can be done, providing extremely useful information in the workup of tailbone pain.

## CT Scans (Computerized Tomography Scans)

CT scans (computerized tomography scans) can provide excellent detail of the skeleton (bones). CT scans also show some details of "soft tissue structures" (body tissues other than bone).

CT scans obtain body images in slices, similar to the way that a block of meat or cheese in a delicatessen could be cut into thin slices. The block of meat or cheese could be sliced from top to bottom, or left to right, or from front to back. Similarly, the CT scan can obtain images that represent slices of the human body from top to bottom, or left to right, or from front to back. Each image shows only the body structures within that slice. Images create a series, or stack, of slices.

- Slices that separate the body from top to bottom (such as slicing the body into an upper half and lower half) are called "axial" slices.

- Slices that separate right from left (slicing the body into a right half and a left half) are called "sagittal" slices.

- Slices that separate front from back (slicing the body into a front half and a back half) are called "coronal" slices.

The combination of axial, sagittal and coronal slices allows the physician to view the human anatomy from multiple angles, or perspectives.

## Problems with CT Scans for Coccyx Pain

The first problem with CT scans for coccyx pain is that most CT scans do not adequately include the coccyx. Some CT scans focus too high up to include the coccyx, such as abdominal CT scans, lumbar CT scans and lumbosacral CT scans. Other CT scans focus too far in front, such as typical pelvic CT scans. Pelvic CT scans generally focus on the organs within the pelvis, such as the urinary bladder, and the male and female reproductive organs (including the female cervix, uterus, and ovaries).

Looking at those pelvic organs can be important since cancer at any of these sites can be a source of pelvic pain. But the standard CT scans often fail to adequately show the coccyx, which is unacceptable in a patient whose primary symptom is coccyx pain. The solution is to have the radiology technician perform additional views (slices), specifically doing sagittal slices at the midline. These types of slices essentially show what the body would look like if cut in half into right and left sides. This usually shows far more detail at the coccyx than a typical pelvic CT scan does.

Another helpful approach to improve the images obtained is for the CT scan to be performed in a more high tech way including "3-D reconstruction." The 3-D (three-dimensional) reconstruction produces images that the physician can rotate on the computer screen in order to see the anatomy from different angles, or points of view.

Another problem with pelvic CT scans is the radiation that the patient is being exposed to. CT scans have become increasingly known as a source of medical radiation that can increase your risk of later developing cancer. This is particularly a concern for pelvic CT scans, since the radiation is being delivered to the male and female reproductive organs, the colon, and other organs in that area, and these are areas already prone to developing cancer. Thus, CT scans can be important and helpful medical tests, but they do carry some risks.

## MRI (Magnetic Resonance Imaging)

An MRI takes images in slices, similar to CT scans (that is, axial, sagittal, and coronal slices). MRI tests are more expensive than CT scans, so insurance companies often make it more difficult for patients to have an MRI. But an MRI has three significant advantages over a CT scan in the workup of patients with tailbone pain.

1. Unlike a CT scan, an MRI does not expose the patient to radiation. This is particularly important in the pelvic region, since radiation here would be delivered to the male and female reproductive organs, potentially putting the patient at increased risk for cancer at those sites.

2. An MRI is often superior to CT scanning in assessing for fluid. An MRI typically includes a set of "T2" images, where fluid such as water shows up bright. This is extremely helpful if looking for inflammation. Just as inflammation causes swelling (fluid) to accumulate at a sprained ankle, dislocated finger, or fractured toe, there is often similar inflammation at a site of coccygeal sprain, dislocation or fracture. An MRI's T2 images can often detect such inflammation. These MRI images can also detect fluid within sites of infection, including bone infection (osteomyelitis) or a nearby abscess (a collection of pus).

3. MRIs are often superior to CT scans at assessing the "soft tissue" (non-bone) structures within the pelvis. This is particularly helpful in screening for whether your tailbone pain might be coming from cancer or other abnormality within your pelvic organs.

## Difficulties with an MRI

Although an MRI is a fantastic test for patients with tailbone pain, there are some challenges to proper MRI testing. The first hurdle is having the MRI images *actually include the tailbone*. This may sound simple enough, but practically every week patients come to me for consultation, bringing MRI studies that were done for their tailbone pain but failed to include the tailbone at all. It is crazy but true!

A main reason for this problem is that the standard MRI studies done for the lower back and pelvis fail to adequately include the tailbone. Most low back pain is in the lumbar region, up around the belt line. So typical MRI testing for back pain focuses on the lumbar spine ("lumbar" MRI or "lumbosacral" MRI) and does not include images down low enough to show the coccyx. Meanwhile, pelvic MRIs are commonly done for assessing structures near the front of the pelvis (such as the male and female reproductive organs), so they do not include images far back enough to show the coccyx.

Often, the solution is for the physician to specifically order a "pelvic MRI" with explicit directions that the MRI radiology technician should perform "thin section midline sagittal images of the coccyx." The idea of "thin" sections essentially means there will be thin image slices obtained. This is similar to the way that your local delicatessen can set its slicing machine to cut the meats or cheeses into slices that are either thicker or thinner. This is important since thin midline slices help ensure that a good image is obtained of the tailbone. The coccyx is a relatively thin structure, and if the slices are not done thinly (close together), it is possible that one slice (image) will be too far to the right of the coccyx but the very next slice will be too far to the left of the coccyx. In that case, the coccyx would be "skipped over," resulting in an image (slice) at each side of the coccyx but no image that fully shows the coccyx.

## Vitamin E Capsule During MRI

Using a single vitamin E capsule can help you to get the proper MRI done and the proper attention from the radiologist. How? The MRI orders can explicitly ask that the radiology technician use a vitamin E capsule, or other MRI-compatible marker, to be taped to the skin over the site of pain. This marker helps the radiology technicians to make sure that they specifically include that body region in the MRI images that are obtained. Further, it draws the attention of the radiologist who will read your MRI, minimizing the chances that he/she will overlook abnormalities in the underlying coccyx. It also helps the treating physician to focus in on the painful area (your coccyx) when he/she is later reviewing the images with you. This is important since many treating physicians may not have sufficient experience looking at coccyx MRI images. Lastly, the skin marker helps empower you (the patient) to be able to look at your own images and see how the site you have marked as painful matches up with your own underlying body anatomy.

## After Your MRI: Get It, Review It, Keep It, Share It.

After your MRI has been completed, it is important for you to make sure that your treating physician receives and review a copy of the official, typed radiology report from the radiologist who read the images. You should generally review these results in person with your treating physician during an office visit, so that any questions or concerns can be addressed. You should also obtain a copy of the written report yourself, to review, save and share with your other treating physicians. Often, a pelvic MRI may reveal findings unrelated to the coccyx, such as abnormalities within the prostate, uterus or ovaries. You should be sure to share those results with your treating primary care physician, urologist, gynecologist, or other appropriate physician depending on where the abnormality was seen. The abnormality could potentially be an underlying malignancy, and prompt evaluation and treatment for cancer can be life-saving.

In addition to obtaining the typed radiology report, you should obtain a copy of your actual MRI images. Most modern MRI facilities will provide this on a computer CD, either for free or at minimal cost. You can then make copies of the computer CD and share the images with your treating physicians.

## "MRI Finger-Pointing Test"

Years ago, I came up with the term "MRI finger-pointing test" as a tip for people who lived too far away to come for evaluation in my office. People with tailbone pain would find me through medical research articles that I had published, and they would reach out to me saying they had tailbone pain but that their MRI had been normal. Since I generally can't give explicit medical advice to people I have not evaluated in person, my tip would be that they ask their own local treating physician to show them their MRI images and *ask the physician explicitly point to the coccyx on the images*. Countless times, I have later heard back that this request prompted the treating physician to look at the MRI images and realize that the tailbone had never been included in the images at all! Or, the tailbone was included in the images, but a blatant abnormality had been overlooked by the radiologist.

A similar tip is that you can respond to the paper radiology report by underlining or highlighting every place that refers to the coccyx, tailbone or coccygeal structures. Again, even though your MRI was done primarily for coccyx pain, you may discover that the radiology report never even mentions the appearance of your coccyx. Such a blatant omission is very concerning. This happens far too frequently. The treating physician (or even the patient) can request that the radiologist issue an official addendum explicitly describing the appearance of the coccyx, including any abnormalities. Meanwhile, if your treating physician will not personally review the actual coccyx images with you to double-check whether the radiologist missed anything, then consider finding medical care elsewhere.

## Bone Scans

A triple phase (three phase) bone scan can be done to look for osteomyelitis (bone infection) or cancer. Cancer at the coccyx could be either a primary cancer (cancer that started within the bone) or a metastatic cancer (cancer that started somewhere else and spread to the bone).

Note that this type of bone scan is very different from the bone "density" scan that is done to look for osteoporosis (thinning of the bones, commonly seen in women after menopause). If the test report uses the term bone "density" or "DEXA," then it is a test for osteoporosis, and it is *not* a test for bone infection or bone cancer.

The bone scan done to look for osteomyelitis and cancer is also called skeletal skintigraphy. These bone scans are usually done by the "nuclear medicine" section of a radiology department, so it is sometimes also called a "nuclear medicine bone scan" (to distinguish it from the DEXA bone density scan done to look for osteoporosis). During a nuclear medicine bone scan, a radioactive material is injected into your bloodstream through an intravenous (IV) line. Skeletal images may be obtained while the injection is being given, then repeated shortly afterwards, and then repeated again 3 to 5 hours later. The third set of images (those images done 3 to 5 hours later) are the "third" phase, or set, of images. This is important since it is this third phase which is best at detecting osteomyelitis. Thus, a "single phase" bone scan may give a false reassurance since it may fail to detect a bone cancer that would have been detected by a three-phase (triple phase) bone scan. A bone scan may also detect other bone abnormalities, such as cancer.

## The Lateral View (Side View) of Bone Scans

When the bone scan images are obtained, the standard views look like a snapshot of the human body from the front and from the back. The images will show one or more "hot spots" where more of the nuclear medicine material becomes concentrated. A hot spot is due to that site having increased bone turnover (that is, both destruction of bone and production of bone). A hot spot shows up bright on the bone scan images.

The biggest problem with the traditional front and back views obtained during a typical bone scan is that these views fail to adequately show the coccyx or lower sacrum. The reason for this failure is that the injected nuclear medicine material (tracer) is excreted from your body by the kidneys, and it pools in the urinary bladder prior to urination. On both the front view and the back view, the view of the coccyx and lower sacral overlaps with the view of the urinary bladder. So, all of the radioactive urine sitting within the urinary bladder creates a huge hot spot which acts like a shadow blocking the view of the coccyx and lower sacrum. This means that the standard front and back views would be completely unable to tell if there was any abnormal hot spot at the coccyx or lower sacrum.

The solution to this problem is to add images done from a side view. In the side view, the urinary bladder can be clearly seen at the front of the pelvis, distinctly separate from the sacrum and coccyx at the back of the pelvis. For new patients at my office, I have often reviewed prior bone scans where the patient and treating physician were told (by the radiologist reading the images) that the bone scan was normal, but my review of the images reveals that the symptomatic area (tailbone) was never even seen in any of the imaging studies. Despite having seen this repeatedly for years, I am still always surprised to see that the specific indication (reason) for doing the test is listed as tailbone pain and yet the images include almost all other bones in the body, *except* for the tailbone!

Yes, the *one* area where the person is having pain is the *only* area in the entire body that is *not* clearly seen on the images! This insanity would be laughable except that the patient is meanwhile still suffering in pain, while the patient and treating doctor are being misled into thinking that the radiologist has properly seen the painful area. Again, if your treating physician is unwilling to review the actual coccyx images with you (to make sure that the radiologist did not miss anything), then you should consider obtaining your medical care elsewhere.

## Bloodwork and Miscellaneous Tests

Bloodwork is not routinely needed or done in the diagnostic workup for most patients with tailbone pain. However, in some cases there may be a specific concern which bloodwork may answer. For example, if there is concern that the tailbone pain is part of a wider distribution of joint problems, such as rheumatoid arthritis, ankylosing spondylitis, or Lyme disease, then bloodwork can be done to check for these.

If there is a concern that you may have a tuberculosis (TB) infection of the coccyx (for example, if you have been in a part of the world where tuberculosis is common), then a PPD skin test can be done to check for exposure to TB. If the PPD skin test is positive, it can be followed by x-rays of the lungs to check for pulmonary tuberculosis. In this or other cases of suspected infection, a biopsy of the tailbone can be removed and sent for microbiology culturing. The cultures are grown to show what bugs (microorganisms or germs) were present in the sample piece of tailbone that was removed during the biopsy.

If problems within the rectum or anus are suspected (for example, if you have pain with bowel movements, blood in your stool, or a family history of rectal cancer), a colonoscopy may be worthwhile to directly visualize the inside of your colon.

### Free Bonus for You

For your free printable form where you can document tests you've had done for tailbone pain, go to: **TailboneDoctor.com/forms**

CHAPTER 17

# Consultations with Other Medical Specialists

## John's Story

What seems like pain at the tailbone may actually be a symptom coming from something else. John's pain in the tailbone region could not be reproduced by pressing externally along the back of the tailbone upon physical examination. This was odd, since most people with tailbone pain have their symptoms brought on by such direct pressure. We wondered whether deeper structures might be causing his pain. He had a family history of colon cancer, so we sent him for consultation with a gastroenterologist (a GI doctor). A colonoscopy revealed colon cancer, which was discovered early enough to be treated successfully with a small, local surgery to remove the tumor. So, although he had self-reported as "tailbone pain," we had looked further. If we had not, then we probably would not have diagnosed his colon cancer until it was too late. The cancer would have spread throughout the body, with potentially deadly consequences.

John's story, and those of many like him, demonstrates the importance of screening for various possible sources of tailbone region pain.

The pelvis is a complex body region with structures that include bones, muscles, tendons, ligaments, male or female reproductive organs, the urinary system, and the gastrointestinal system (colon and rectum). So, it should be no surprise that evaluation and treatment of pelvic abnormalities often involves getting

**One challenge, however, is finding a pain management physician who has adequate experience in specifically treating coccydynia.**

input from a variety of different medical specialists, with their different perspectives due to their different areas of expertise.

## Primary Care Physician

Ideally, all patients should have a primary care physician to oversee their overall medical care. This is typically a physician in Internal Medicine or Family Practice, or Pediatrics for children. You should keep your primary care physician (PCP) up-to-date with the results of specialist consultations and tests that have been done. Although consultants, labs and imaging centers can usually send a copy of your reports to the PCP if you request this, it is often better for you to receive these copies yourself and personally bring them to a follow-up visit with your PCP, to ensure that they have been delivered, reviewed and responded to. Working closely with your PCP is one of the cornerstones of good medical care.

## Pain Management Physician

Pain management physicians specialize in treating a wide variety of painful conditions. They often prescribe various types of pain-relieving medications, including nonsteroidal anti-inflammatory drugs (NSAIDs, such as ibuprofen), opioid/narcotic painkillers (such as oxycodone), and medications to relieve nerve pain. They also often perform a variety of injections to relieve pain. These injections may include steroid injections, nerve blocks, and nerve destruction injections (ablation).

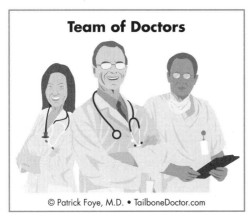

**Team of Doctors**

© Patrick Foye, M.D. • TailboneDoctor.com

One challenge, however, is finding a pain management physician who has adequate experience in specifically treating coccydynia. To assess for this, you may wish to call your local pain management physician's office and ask the receptionist whether the physician specifically treats "coccydynia" or performs "ganglion Impar injections." If the receptionist responds by sounding confused, hesitant, uncertain, or unfamiliar with these terms (or if you need to explain what those terms mean), then most likely the physician's practice is rarely, if ever, providing this subspecialty type of medical care. (Most likely that physician group rarely treats tailbone pain.) A brief call to the receptionist will often tell you what you need to know.

## Pelvic Floor Physical Therapist

The pelvic floor includes a collection of muscles, tendons and ligaments that help to support the internal organs of the pelvis. They act like a hammock or sling, holding up the pelvic organs and keeping them from sagging or falling down toward the ground. Just as a hammock has an attachment site on each end, so too does the pelvic floor have an attachment area at the front of the pelvis and at the back of the pelvis. The attachment at the front of the pelvis includes the pubic bones, just above the genitals. The attachment at the back of the pelvis includes the coccyx. Some patients with focal coccyx pain and coccyx abnormalities have little or no additional problems with their pelvic floor. Other coccyx patients do indeed have extensive additional pain, spasm, and other problems within their pelvic floor.

Patients with substantial pelvic floor dysfunction should strongly consider seeing a physical therapist (PT) who has special training in this area. Most physical therapists do not have much experience or expertise in treating pelvic floor problems. Fortunately, however, increasingly there are physical therapists specializing in pelvic floor rehabilitation. These PTs have training and experience in doing internal examination. This involves having the PT place a few fingers inside your vagina or anus to feel for focal areas of tenderness within specific muscles and other structures. They can also use their internal fingers to massage and stretch the levator ani muscles, coccygeus muscles, or other sites that may be causing pain.

For patients who have pain diffusely throughout the pelvic floor or genital region (often associated with pain during sex, or irritability of the urinary bladder or bowels), finding a local physical therapist with expertise in pelvic floor dysfunction can be a great step forward toward recovery.

For my patients at the Tailbone Pain Center, if the problem is focal to the coccyx (such as a coccygeal bone spur), then I typically concentrate my initial treatment at the coccyx. But if there are substantial symptoms throughout the pelvic floor, then it is certainly worthwhile to try to find a pelvic floor physical therapist in the patient's locality. Similarly, many pelvic floor physical therapists who find a coccyx abnormality that is failing to respond to therapy often refer those patients for evaluation at our Tailbone Pain Center.

As with many areas in life and in medicine, a team approach often works best.

## Gynecologist, for Female Reproductive Organs

Female reproductive organs can be a source of many abnormalities resulting in pelvic pain. Cancer and other abnormalities can occur at the cervix, uterus or ovaries. Pain from these sites can radiate (travel) to include the tailbone region. Female patients with tailbone pain should see their local obstetrician/gynecologist and explicitly report these symptoms. A careful history and physical examination can help assess whether any of the symptoms are coming from problems within the female reproductive organs.

Some gynecologists specialize in treating pelvic floor pain and other pelvic pain syndromes.

Discussions with the obstetrician/gynecologist are also important if the woman with tailbone pain is considering having a baby. Plans should be made for optimizing the mother's health, and minimizing her pain, during both pregnancy and delivery. Tailbone pain and pregnancy are covered in further detail in a later chapter of this book. (See Chapter 27: *Pregnancy, Childbirth and Tailbone Pain*.)

## Gastroenterologist, for Colonoscopy

Your rectum is the lowest part of the large intestine (colon) and is the site where stool collects prior to it being pushed out through the anus during a bowel movement. Your rectum is located just in front of the tailbone. Rectal cancer (as well as other colon cancers) can cause pain in the tailbone region. To screen for cancers of the colon, current public health recommendations include a routine colonoscopy starting when you are 50-years-old, or sooner if you have a family history of colon cancer or have any symptoms of the lower gastrointestinal tract (such as blood in the stool or pain with bowel movements).

During a colonoscopy, the physician uses a video camera on the tip of a flexible tube that is inserted through the anus into the colon. Abnormal or suspicious areas can be biopsied, with the tissue sample then sent for pathology evaluation to see whether it is cancer. There are also multiple non-cancer causes of anal pain and rectal pain, most of which are treatable. These include hemorrhoids, anal fissures (tears), perianal abscess, and proctitis (inflammation of the rectum and anus). As with most medical conditions, the earlier the diagnosis and treatment are begun, the better the outcome for the patient.

## Urologist, for Urinary Problems

Patients who have significant symptoms of their urinary system should consider seeing a urologist. Your symptoms could include frequent urination, pain or burning during urination, inability to control the urinary bladder (urinary incontinence), or repeated episodes of urinary tract infections. You may have a diagnosis of interstitial cystitis (IC). Interstitial cystitis can be notoriously difficult to diagnose and treat.

Men with pain or other symptoms in the male genital region (penis, scrotum, or testicles) should also consider evaluation by a urologist.

## Oncologist, for Cancer

Patients with a history of cancer should follow through with whatever recommended monitoring or follow-up plan has been recommended by the physician who treated that cancer. Often this is an oncologist, which is a physician who specializes in treating cancers. In other cases, the responsible physician may be a specialist in the organ system where the malignancy occurred, such as a gynecologist for cancer of the female reproductive system, or a urologist for male prostate cancer. One reason to make the responsible physician aware of the tailbone pain is that this may be a signal that the prior cancer has returned and has spread to the tailbone.

## Orthopedic Surgeon, for Coccygectomy

In the rare cases where coccyx pain fails to respond adequately to nonsurgical treatment (including cushions, medications by mouth, or various types of tailbone injections), it may be worthwhile to consider surgical removal of the coccyx (coccygectomy). Probably one out of every 30 or 40 patients who I see for tailbone pain ends up failing to get adequate relief from nonsurgical treatment and therefore ends up seeing a surgeon for consultation for possible coccygectomy. In these cases, it is important (and often challenging) to find a surgeon who is experienced at performing this uncommon surgery. As with all surgeries, there are many potential risks and benefits.

Further details regarding surgery to remove the tailbone are included in a later chapter. (See Chapter 25: *Coccygectomy: Surgical Removal of the Tailbone.*)

### Free Bonus for You

For your free printable form where you can document and track your consults with medical specialists, go to: **TailboneDoctor.com/forms**

# PART TWO

# Treatments to Relieve Your Tailbone Pain

## In This Section

**18** Treatments for Tailbone Pain:
Overview ............................ 141

**19** Avoid Worsening Your
Tailbone Pain ......................... 145

**20** Cushions for Tailbone Pain ........ 151

**21** Medications for Tailbone Pain ..... 159

**22** Manipulation of the Coccyx ....... 169

**23** Exercise and Tailbone Pain......... 175

**24** Injections for Tailbone Pain......... 181

**25** Coccygectomy: Surgical Removal
of the Tailbone ...................... 195

# CHAPTER 18

# Treatments for Tailbone Pain:
## Overview

Many people feel frustrated and hopeless when their local doctors incorrectly tell them that there are no treatments available for tailbone pain. In actuality, there are a wide variety of treatments available, and these are helpful for the vast majority of people with tailbone pain.

**There are a wide variety of treatments available, and these are helpful for the vast majority of people with tailbone pain.**

Upcoming chapters in this book will cover these various treatments. The chapters generally follow the sequence from the simplest approaches to the most complex. The first topic covered is avoiding exacerbating factors, then medications taken by mouth, followed by medications given by local injection, and finally surgical removal of the tailbone (coccygectomy).

This sequence of treatment options is not carved in stone. The sequence needs to be individualized to each specific patient. For example, patients with stomach ulcers, liver problems, kidney disease, or irritable bowel syndrome might have substantial difficulty tolerating many of the pain medications taken by mouth, because they can cause side effects throughout those areas. Those patients may be better off skipping or minimizing the medications by mouth and instead just have medications given focally at the site of pain, by a small injection at the tailbone. Surgical removal of the tailbone (coccygectomy) is typically only recommended in the uncommon cases where most or all of the other treatment options have already been tried yet have failed to give adequate relief. However, in the rare cases where the tailbone pain is caused by a cancer, then surgical removal of the malignancy would often be the prompt next step. Physical therapy might be appropriate at any stage of the treatment, depending on the specific diagnosis and whether the tailbone pain has resulted in additional pain in nearby muscles and tendons.

Patient preference, of course, plays a large role in the sequence of treatment options tried. Some patients are reluctant to take oral medications because they do not like the idea of these chemicals traveling throughout their body, even if they are helpful for the pain. They may prefer the human, hands-on touch provided by a physical therapist. Alternatively, some patients may find the idea of a physical therapist's or chiropractor's internal treatment (with one or more of the clinician's fingers placed inside the patient's vagina or rectum) to be something the patient is squeamish about or considers too invasive.

Even the patient's hometown geography can play a significant factor. Many patients are limited in the number and type of clinicians who have expertise in treating tailbone pain in the patient's local geographic region. A patient who lives within traveling distance of our Tailbone Pain Center may be content to return once every year or two for a repeat injection, if the pain returns. All of this varies from patient to patient.

The subsequent chapters will provide information on the various treatments, which can then be individualized for the specific patient with tailbone pain.

CHAPTER 19

# Avoid Worsening Your Tailbone Pain

## Ashley's Story

Every day for Ashley seemed to revolve around constantly figuring out how she could avoid worsening her tailbone pain. She carried her tailbone cushion with her everywhere. She generally stood up instead of sitting. She even obtained a special sit-stand desk that allowed her to alternate between sitting and standing while using her computer at work. She avoided horseback riding, water slides, roller coasters, and certain yoga poses. Ashley had a small bone spur on her lower coccyx. As long as she avoided flaring up her tailbone, on most days she had little or no pain at all, without any need for medications, injections or surgery. By avoiding exacerbating activities, she dramatically improved her quality of life.

## Sitting

The first and most natural reaction when something is painful is to avoid doing what makes the pain worse. Tailbone pain is typically worst with sitting and especially with sitting leaning partway backward. Thus, you may naturally try to avoid sitting and particularly avoid sitting in a slightly reclined (backward leaning) position.

You may try to avoid sitting by standing instead. Obviously this standing approach works better with some jobs than with others. Some workers are able to perform their job duties while standing at a drafting table instead of sitting down at a regular desk. Some people will use a sit-stand desk, which allows the desktop height to be raised or lowered intermittently throughout the workday, so

**Tailbone pain is typically worst with sitting and especially with sitting leaning partway backward.**

that the person can alternate between sitting and standing, as tolerated. Raising and lowering these sit-stand workstations can require the manual use of a crank handle, or (more conveniently) they can be electrically powered.

Unfortunately, many jobs and situations do not easily allow individuals to personally control when they sit or stand throughout the workday. Most of us need to remain seated while we drive to and from work, school or errands. Bus drivers and taxi cab drivers must sit while driving. Pilots and passengers must remain seated during most of an airline flight. Business people would generally find it awkward to stand throughout a business meeting when their clients and coworkers in the meeting are all sitting down. In a court room trial, lawyers or jurors who stood throughout the case might be considered disruptive. A meal out at a restaurant almost always requires sitting down to eat at a table.

Another limitation against just standing throughout the day is that many patients have other musculoskeletal conditions (at sites other than the tailbone) that would be aggravated by prolonged standing. For example, you may have arthritis in your knees or lower back, or degenerative disc problems within your lower back. These may make prolonged standing problematic. Also, you may simply lack the physical stamina or endurance to stand throughout the majority of the day.

Thus, while avoiding sitting is a natural first approach in patients with tailbone pain, sitting is often unavoidable.

If you must sit despite tailbone pain, you can at least alter your sitting posture to minimize your pain. You may find that your tailbone pain while sitting is less if you sit leaning forward or leaning toward either the right or left side. These positions decrease how much of your body weight is pushing down through the tailbone and onto the chair or other sitting surface. Some people are flexible enough that they can bend a leg back such that one of their feet can then be sat upon by one buttock, thereby elevating that buttock and again decreasing the coccygeal weight-bearing.

You may find that some sitting surfaces are worse than others. Tailbone pain may be exacerbated by sitting on a harder surface for some patients and sitting on a softer surface for other patients. You may find that certain couches or chairs exacerbate your tailbone pain much more than others do. Try to learn to avoid the more problematic seats.

## Recreational Exacerbation

Some recreational activities are known to cause or exacerbate tailbone pain. For example, cycling, horseback riding, roller coasters, snowmobiles, jet skis, and waterslides are known to physically involve forceful or repetitive bouncing upon the buttock and tailbone region. Many patients with tailbone pain decide that the risk of exacerbation from these types of activities is simply not worth the enjoyment that the activities provide.

Some activities only cause trauma to the tailbone if you fall, but the activity may have an inherently increased risk of falls. Examples include rollerblading, ice skating, and certain martial

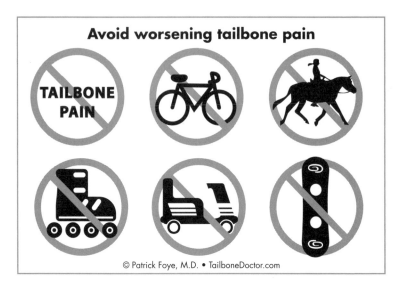

arts. You need to personally evaluate the likelihood of falls and the likelihood that such a fall would worsen your pain. You can then compare your personal enjoyment of the activity with the potential risk for exacerbation, and make an informed decision of whether to continue taking these risks.

You may decide that your enjoyment of certain specific activities is not enough to be worth risking exacerbation. So you may avoid the activities even if the tailbone pain has been gone for years.

Alternatively, appropriate diagnosis and treatment of your tailbone pain may allow you to fully resume all previous activities. Unfortunately, sometimes even after treatment provides 100 percent relief for years, the pain may return if you resume an activity that puts substantial pressure on your tailbone. So, each patient must decide how his/her enjoyment of a given activity is balanced by the potential risk for exacerbation of tailbone pain.

## Clothing That May Worsen Tailbone Pain

Some people with tailbone pain find that their pain is worsened by clothing that causes direct pressure on the coccyx. For example, denim jeans with a thick, prominent seam over the sacrum and coccyx may worsen tailbone pain, especially if the clothing is tight. Similarly, thong underwear can cause direct pressure onto the coccyx. Individuals whose tailbone pain is worsened by clothing may benefit from switching to clothing that is slightly looser or has less prominent seams over the coccyx.

## Disability Forms and Other Restrictions

Some patients with tailbone pain ask whether they are medically "allowed" to perform a given physical activity. For most coccydynia patients, this mainly comes down to what your symptoms allow you to tolerate, rather then a strict mandate dictated by the treating physician. There are, however, times when the treating physician can document for you the tailbone condition and the expected, common, resultant limitations for purposes of documenting activities such as work status, school modifications, travel restrictions, or jury duty limitations.

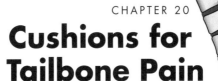

# CHAPTER 20

# Cushions for Tailbone Pain

## Robert's Story

Although Robert's primary physician had recommended a circular doughnut cushion, he found that sitting on it was awkward and actually made his tailbone pain feel worse. He incorrectly assumed that all cushions for tailbone pain were about the same, so he resigned himself to the idea that such cushions are useless. We recommended that he instead try a wedge cushion. Robert found that it was vastly more helpful than the doughnut cushion. While it was not a cure, the wedge cushion dramatically improved his comfort while sitting. Using the cushion, Robert was once again able to sit long enough to get through business meetings, his work commute, and even an occasional airline flight.

A common initial treatment for patients with tailbone pain is to use a cushion. The goal of the cushion is to decrease the pressure placed upon the coccyx during sitting, and thus decrease the pain.

There are a wide variety of cushions available, each with advantages and disadvantages. In general, these cushions are portable enough that you can easily carry your cushion from home, to your car, work, school, and restaurants. Some cushions have a strap that serves as a handle to make carrying the cushion more convenient. The cushions are relatively inexpensive

**Wedge cushions are typically superior to donut (ring) cushions for patients with tailbone pain.**

($10 to $50, plus shipping costs), so you may find it easier to just buy a few cushions and keep one at each location where you sit throughout the day. It makes sense to try one cushion first to make sure that it works well for you, prior to purchasing many of that same type.

## Doughnut Cushions, Ring Cushions

Many patients with tailbone pain are told to try sitting on a doughnut cushion (ring cushion). These cushions form a circular ring with a hole in the center. The general idea is that you are supposed to sit in such a way that the tailbone is above the hole in the center of the cushion, so that the tailbone is not weight-bearing while you are sitting.

Although these ring (doughnut) cushions are commonly recommended to patients, they are not the best cushions to use for tailbone pain. First of all, many patients find these ring cushions to be uncomfortable. Some patients have a difficult time getting the positioning just right. You may find it tough to predict or figure out exactly where your coccyx is located in relationship to the hole in the cushion. Secondly, some patients feel that the circular pressure caused by the inner edges of the ring create a noose-like effect on the coccyx and anal region. Thirdly, because the cushion makes a full ring, or circle, that means that the back-most portion of the ring can create pressure on the upper coccyx or lower sacrum. This pressure can be uncomfortable if you have arthritis or instability at the upper coccyx. For all of these reasons, the ring cushion, while helpful for a few coccyx patients, may actually worsen the tailbone pain for many other coccyx patients.

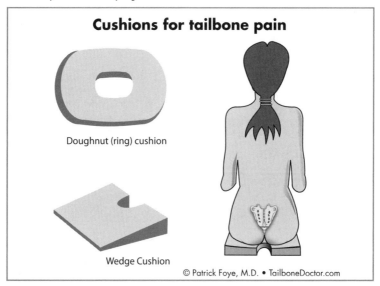

## Cushions for tailbone pain

Doughnut (ring) cushion

Wedge Cushion

© Patrick Foye, M.D. • TailboneDoctor.com

## Wedge Cushions

Wedge cushions are typically superior to donut (ring) cushions for patients with tailbone pain. The term "wedge cushion" generally refers to two important features about these cushions. First, the cushion is typically shaped overall like a square but has a wedge-shaped cutout at the back. The shape would be similar to a square cake where someone had then cut out a triangle-shaped piece of cake, causing that wedge-shaped piece to be missing from the back of the cake. When you sit on this cushion, your tailbone hovers up above the open wedge space, so that your tailbone does not receive direct pressure from your body weight or the seat below. Unlike the doughnut (ring) cushion, the wedge cushion has no back wall, so the wedge cushion does not inadvertently cause painful pressure onto the back of the upper coccyx or lower sacrum.

The second feature of a "wedge" cushion is that many of them will have an overall "tilt" to the cushion from back to front. Looking at the cushion from the side, the back of the cushion is taller than the front of the cushion, so that the side view looks like a wedge. When you sit on the cushion, this slight incline tends to have you tilt slightly forward at your pelvis, which is a sitting position that typically helps relieve tailbone pain.

## Neck Pillows

Airplane travelers and mass transit commuters may be familiar with U-shaped neck pillows that people use to keep their head upright if they fall asleep during a trip. Many people with tailbone pain have found that they can sit on these pillows and relieve their tailbone pain if they turn the U-shape around so that the opening is at the back (under the tailbone).

Note that an inflatable (air-filled) neck pillow is unlikely to be strong enough or durable enough to support your body weight while sitting on it. However, the neck pillows that are filled with a bean-bag type of beads can often provide adequate support and durability.

## Boppy, for Breastfeeding Mothers

Many mothers who are breastfeeding are familiar with using a "Boppy"® cushion. This is a U-shaped cushion which the mother typically places around her abdomen to help support the baby that is breastfeeding. Basically, this cushion holds the baby sideways at the appropriate height, or level, for the baby to feed from the mother's breast. This can be extremely helpful, so that the mother does not need to use her arms to hold the baby up throughout the entire breastfeeding session.

Many women with tailbone pain have found that the Boppy cushion can be helpful at relieving tailbone pain while sitting. The cushion can be placed on the chair with the opening of the U-shape being at the back, so that when you sit on it your tailbone will be above the opening.

## Custom-Made Cushions

Over the years, I have seen many custom-made cushions and seats that patients with coccyx pain have brought with them when they come to our Tailbone Pain Center. I have seen various toilet seats, pool noodles, and plywood covered with padding (such as various types of fluffy stuffing, beads, Styrofoam). Sometimes these are covered with beautiful designer fabrics. Some look like works of art!

## Cushion Firmness versus Softness

How firm should a tailbone cushion be? Or, how soft should it be? The answer is usually to avoid extremes at either side of the spectrum.

Also, each individual is different. So different people will prefer different cushions. Just as in the fairytale where Goldilocks tried the bears' beds to find which was "too hard," "too soft," or "just right," you may need to try different coccyx cushions to find the one that is best for you.

Many cushions are too soft. If the cushion lacks adequate firmness or support, then the person's body weight will compress the cushion, preventing the necessary support. So, the cushion initially looks like it would support your lower buttocks and keep your tailbone hovering in midair an inch above the chair. But if the cushion is too soft then your buttocks compress and flatten out the cushion to the point where your tailbone may touch the chair. The goal of that cushion has been defeated. Sometimes the cushion starts out being too soft, straight from the manufacturer. Other times a cushion that worked fine initially may soften over many months of use, becoming less effective and less helpful.

Sometimes a cushion is too firm. Some patients have even used a brick or a text book under each of the two buttocks, so that the midline tailbone will hover without touching the chair. This is highly effective at keeping the tailbone from making contact with the chair, but may cause excessive pressure on the areas where the hard support is making contact with the body.

For example, the hard support (or cushion) may cause excessive pressure on the ischial "sit bones" at the bottom of each buttock. This can result in ischial bursitis, which is characterized by local pain and inflammation at the lower right or left buttocks.

A cushion or support that is too firm may also put excessive pressure at the back of the upper thigh. The largest nerve to the leg (the sciatic nerve) passes through this area and can be compressed. So a cushion that is too firm may cause excessive pressure on the sciatic nerve, resulting in feelings of pain, numbness or tingling down into one or both legs. Patients report that their legs feel like they "fall asleep." Sometimes sitting far forward onto the front edge of a seat (again, to avoid putting pressure on the tailbone) can result in this same type of sciatic nerve irritation.

## Individualized Choice of Cushions

A person who is particularly heavy will compress the cushion material more than someone who is petite. So, the heavier person may require a firmer cushion. Alternatively, the person experiencing sciatic nerve compression at the back of the upper thigh might need a softer cushion.

## Custom Toilet Seat

Some patients with tailbone pain report that sitting is always painful except for sitting on a toilet seat. Some patients have told me the pain got to the point where they started doing their computer work while sitting on the toilet, with a folding table in front of them to hold up their laptop. A number of my patients decided that the toilet seat was so helpful that they started to carry a toilet seat with them for sitting at home or at work. Using a clean, new one and disguising it with some fabric cover may help avoid making your family and coworkers squeamish.

## Hard, Thin Plastic Shell

Maybe this one can't rightfully be called a "cushion" so much as a portable sitting surface. There is at least one manufacturer that makes a thin, hard plastic shell that cradles the buttocks while sitting. The plastic shell has an indentation or bump out area where the tailbone would normally contact the sitting surface. The indentation creates a space so that the tailbone does not make contact, so there is less pressure on the tailbone and therefore there is less pain while sitting.

The hard plastic shell is very lightweight and thus very portable. It is very durable, since there is no soft material to wear down or become more compressed over time. Many patients with tailbone pain report less pain with sitting on a hard surface rather than a soft surface, and the hard plastic shell essentially provides you with a hard surface to use wherever you are sitting. So even if you need to sit on a soft chair or couch, using the hard shell can provide a more rigid support.

## Which Cushion Is Best?

Simply put, the best cushion is the one that works best for you. There is no one brand or style of cushion that will work best for every person with tailbone pain. If the first cushion that you try is not helpful, try a different type. If a cushion worked really well for you but became worn down and unhelpful many months or years later, replace it with a new one of the same type. If you find the "perfect cushion" for you, buy a few of them, so that you can keep one at your computer desk at work, another at your computer at home, and perhaps another at your dining room chair or in your car.

## Don't Throw Away Your Cushion

If local tailbone injections or other treatments provide 100 percent relief, consider continuing to use the cushion, to minimize any chance of the pain coming back.

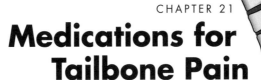

# CHAPTER 21

# Medications for Tailbone Pain

**Melissa's Story**

As a working mother, Melissa was frustrated that the pain medicines prescribed by her primary care physician for her tailbone pain made her too groggy to fully perform her work and home activities. She felt like the medications put her mind into a brain fog. It made no sense to her that her focal problem at the tailbone was being treated mainly with medications that traveled mainly to all other areas throughout her body. Melissa was worried about medication side-effects in her stomach, liver and kidneys. By providing medication locally at the tailbone by a small focal injection, we were able to provide excellent relief and remove her need for taking any pain medications by mouth. Melissa was a new person.

Tailbone pain can be treated with a variety of medications. This chapter provides an overview of medications used to treat tailbone pain. You will discover many categories and specific examples of pain-relieving medications that can be taken by mouth, or applied to the skin, or even sprayed into the nose.

## NSAIDs: Nonsteroidal Anti-Inflammatory Drugs

### Reasons to Use NSAIDs

Many widely used pain-relieving (analgesic) medications are NSAIDs (nonsteroidal anti-inflammatory drugs). Excessive inflammation is a common problem at many sites of musculoskeletal pain and injury. Just as when you injure or sprain your ankle and there is an inflammatory response that causes swelling, so too is there an inflammatory response when you injure or sprain your tailbone.

**One problem with taking medicines by mouth for a focal, localized problem like tailbone pain is that only a tiny amount of the medication will act locally at your site of pain.**

For your swollen ankle, you might keep your ankle elevated and wrap it with an elastic sleeve or bandage. You can't do those things for your tailbone. But you can use NSAIDs for both your injured ankle and for your injured coccyx.

The three main beneficial effects of NSAIDs are to decrease inflammation, decrease pain, and decrease fevers. The first two out of three apply to tailbone pain: decreasing inflammation and decreasing pain.

### Availability and Examples of NSAIDs

One reason why NSAIDs are so commonly used is that they are widely available. You can obtain many different NSAIDs either over the counter or with a physician's prescription. Common examples include aspirin (Bufferin®, Ecotrin®, Excedrin®), celecoxib (Celebrex®), diclofenac (Cataflam®, Voltaren®, Arthrotec®), etodolac (Lodine®), ibuprofen (Advil®, Motrin®, Nuprin®), indomethacine (Indocin®), meloxicam (Mobic®), nabumetone (Relafen®), naproxen (Naprosyn®, Naprelan®), naproxen sodium (Aleve®, Anaprox®), and many others.

For many of these NSAIDs, a physician's prescription provides a prescription strength that is typically a stronger pain reliever than the over-the-counter version. For example, over-the-counter ibuprofen is a 200 mg tablet, while prescription strength ibuprofen is typically 600 mg or 800 mg (three to four times stronger). The prescription strength is typically much more effective at relieving pain, and far more effective at reducing inflammation, than the over-the-counter version. But the higher dose results in a higher likelihood of side effects.

## Side Effects of NSAIDs

NSAIDs can be terrific medications for relieving pain and inflammation, but unfortunately they have many side effects.

Side effects of the gastrointestinal system (stomach and intestines) are common and problematic. NSAIDs can cause painful irritation of the stomach lining, known as gastritis. NSAIDs can cause ulceration of the stomach and intestines, including bleeding ulcers. This type of internal bleeding from NSAIDs results in thousands of hospitalizations per year. Many people die due to unrecognized internal blood loss. There are at least three causes of this:

- NSAIDs directly irritate the stomach lining.

- NSAIDs inhibit a particular chemical (prostaglandin) that is needed to protect the stomach lining.

- NSAIDs are blood thinners, so once someone starts bleeding (from a stomach ulcer) unfortunately the blood fails to clot to stop the bleeding.

The blood thinning side effect can create problems beyond the stomach and intestines. You may bruise more easily even with minor trauma. You may bleed inside your brain (called a hemorrhagic stroke, which can be catastrophic, even deadly).

The blood thinning side effect of NSAIDs is even more dangerous if you are already on another blood thinner, such as warfarin (Coumadin®), enoxaparin sodium (Lovenox®), or ticlopidine (Ticlid®).

NSAIDs also cause a wide variety of other side effects, including kidney damage, elevated blood pressure (hypertension), and increased risks for strokes and heart attacks.

Because of their side effects, NSAIDs should be avoided (or used with caution) if you are on blood thinners or if you have a history of gastritis, peptic ulcer disease, hiatal hernia, esophagitis, excessive vaginal bleeding, kidney disease, or poorly controlled hypertension.

Overall, NSAIDs can be terrific for relieving pain and inflammation, but they do carry real and significant risks of side effects. Over-the-counter NSAIDs may be appropriate for short-term use if you do not have any medical contraindications.

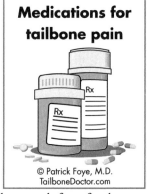

**Medications for tailbone pain**

© Patrick Foye, M.D.
TailboneDoctor.com

One problem with taking medicines by mouth for a focal, localized problem like tailbone pain is that only a tiny amount of the medication will act locally at your site of pain. If you only have a tiny amount of inflammation or pain at your tailbone, then the tiny amount of NSAID that reaches that site may be adequate to provide relief. But if your tailbone pain or inflammation is more substantial, then the oral NSAID might be only minimally helpful, or not at all. Meanwhile, while only a small amount of the ingested NSAID goes to your tailbone, the majority of it goes to the stomach, kidneys, and other body organs where it can cause side effects. This is a big part of why medications given by local injection at the tailbone may be more effective and safer than medications taken by mouth.

## Steroids by Mouth

The term "*non*-steroidal" anti-inflammatory drugs (NSAIDs) correctly implies that there are also "steroidal" anti-inflammatory drugs. Steroids can powerfully decrease inflammation. Common examples of steroids taken by mouth include methylprednisolone (such as Medrol® dose pack) and prednisone.

These anti-inflammatory types of steroids are very different than the anabolic steroids that bodybuilders and athletes have often abused. These anti-inflammatory types of steroids won't help you hit more home runs or become Mr. Universe (sorry, Arnold).

Some people with rheumatoid arthritis and other rheumatologic or immunologic conditions take oral steroids every day for years to decrease their body's overactive inflammatory response. Doctors may also prescribe a short course (several days) of oral steroids for a patient with a short-term inflammatory condition.

Although the oral steroids are often more powerful than non-steroidals at decreasing inflammation, they unfortunately are more difficult for patients to tolerate. Some of the steroid side effects are similar to those seen with nonsteroidals, including gastrointestinal problems such as upset stomach, stomach ulcers, gastritis, and internal bleeding within the stomach or intestines.

Steroids also carry additional risks for side effects rarely seen with nonsteroidals. These include swelling within the feet/ankles, difficulty sleeping, and mental changes such as confusion, anxiety or depression.

As with nonsteroidals, steroids taken by mouth go throughout the body, not just to the site where you need the anti-inflammatory benefit. One solution is to give an anti-inflammatory steroid locally at the inflamed, painful site, by a small local injection. However, there first should be an accurate diagnosis of which specific tailbone joint or site is problematic, with the steroid injection then done under visualization (such as fluoroscopy) to accurately target the problematic site.

## Opioid (Narcotic) Painkillers

Your tailbone pain may be so severe and disruptive to quality of life that opioid (narcotic) painkillers are considered.

A few decades ago, opioid pain killers were mainly only used either for short-term relief after things like fractures or surgeries, or as part of compassionate end-of-life care for dying cancer patients. But nowadays there is increasing understanding that these medications can be helpful for many types of chronic pain that are neither life-threatening nor due to cancer.

Common examples of opioid analgesics include oxycodone (Percocet®, OxyContin®), hydrocodone (Vicodin®, Norco®), fentanyl (Duragesic® patches), hydromorphone (Dilaudid®, Exalgo®), and morphine (Avinza®, MS Contin®).

Opioid analgesics are the most powerful painkillers available. However, they also have substantial and sometimes life-threatening side effects.

The most common side effects of opioid analgesics are sedation and constipation. Sedation may be severe, making you feel tired, sleepy, fatigued, or drained of energy, to the point where you can barely get out of bed. Or the sedation may be more subtle, where you just lack your full vitality for life.

Constipation due to opioids can be severely problematic. Opioids slow down the movement of food and stool within your intestines. As bowel movements become less frequent, your abdomen can feel uncomfortable, full or firm. Stool backed up within your large intestine can cause pressure onto your tailbone, making your tailbone pain even worse. Straining to push out a bowel movement can also make your tailbone pain worse.

Constipation due to opioids can be treated with stool softeners and, much more importantly, with laxatives (which stimulate the bowels to keep moving).

There are various other side effects of opioid painkillers. Psychologically, the sedation or fatigue may cause or worsen depression. These medications can be addictive and can be abused by patients who receive these prescriptions or by others who have access to their medications. Overdose, whether intentional (suicidal) or accidental, can be deadly.

Opioids can depress or slow breathing, which is especially problematic in individuals with pre-existing breathing disorders.

Caution: Opioid addiction can be problematic, especially in people who have a history of prior drug addiction.

Despite these side effects, opioid analgesics can be helpful, when appropriately prescribed and appropriately used.

## Medications for Nerve Pain

Some medications treat nerve pain. These include certain antidepressant medications and anti-seizure medications. Antidepressants used to treat nerve pain include amitriptyline (Elavil®) and duloxetine (Cymbalta®). Anti-seizure medications used to treat nerve pain include gabapentin (Neurontin®, Gralise®) and pregabalin (Lyrica®). Side effects commonly include sedation (fatigue).

Unfortunately, there is no substantial research to support (or refute) using these medications specifically for tailbone pain.

## Nasal Calcitonin

Calcitonin given by nasal spray (into the nose) is sometimes used to treat spinal fractures. Calcitonin is felt to both decrease the fracture pain and improve fracture healing. Specific to coccyx fractures, our landmark study (published in 2014) that we did here at the Tailbone Pain Center showed that patients with coccyx fractures had significant relief while using nasal calcitonin, just one spray in one nostril each day. The most common side effect is nasal irritation, which is minimized by alternating which nostril receives the nasal spray on any given day (that is, one spray into the right nostril on one day followed by the left nostril on the next day).

## Topical Creams or Lotions

There are a number of over-the-counter (non-prescription) and prescription creams and lotions advertised to help relieve pain. These are intended to be rubbed onto areas of sore muscles or over arthritic joints.

Some patients who have tried these for tailbone pain have reported mild relief. But so far no research study has looked at these to show whether they help much for tailbone pain.

In addition to NSAIDs (nonsteroidal anti-inflammatory drugs) taken by mouth, NSAIDs can also be applied to the skin over an area of pain or inflammation. The idea is that instead of having to travel throughout the entire body the medication acts locally just at the site where you need it. Examples include various forms of diclofenac, such as Voltaren gel®, Pennsaid®, and Flector patches®. The patches are difficult to use for tailbone pain since the patches typically need a flat surface to stick to (unlike the "crack" between the two buttocks). The topical gels and creams face the difficulties discussed in the next paragraphs below.

Regarding side effects, I have seen patients suffer from skin irritation and even skin breakdown from applying topical medications to the skin over the tailbone. The skin over the tailbone may be susceptible to these side effects for a number of reasons. The skin over the tailbone doesn't get a chance to "breathe" as well as the skin in most other body regions. Firstly, the skin is in the "crack" in between the right and left buttocks, and each buttock may overlap or extend a bit over the midline skin. This inhibits the skin's ability to "breathe," since it is losing contact with the air. Secondly, we wear clothing over the buttock and pelvic region. The clothing further inhibits the skin's ability to breathe. Thirdly, we typically sit upon the coccyx, meaning that the skin will be compressed some-what against the chair. This further impairs the skin's ability to breathe.

Another problem with topical creams over the tailbone is that the skin there is very close to the anus, so fecal matter from bowel movements may stick to the creams and lotions applied to the skin in that area. This can cause skin irritation and hygiene problems.

**Free Bonus for You**

For your free printable list of medications that decrease tailbone pain, go to: **TailboneDoctor.com/forms**

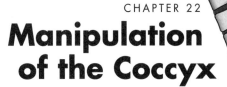

CHAPTER 22

# Manipulation of the Coccyx

## Samantha's Story

Samantha's osteopathic doctor told her that her tailbone was "out of alignment" and that it would feel fine once he moved it back into the proper position. He placed one finger inside her anus and the other behind her tailbone and moved it forward and backward. Although the procedure was painful and awkward for her, she then felt some relief for the next few hours. But the pain came back again and again despite several of these treatments. In Samantha's case, manipulation was not the solution.

Coccyx manipulation, mobilization, or adjustment are hands-on approaches where a health professional intentionally moves your coccygeal bones. This is a type of "manual medicine" technique. Although I do not frequently provide coccyx manipulation at the Tailbone Pain Center, this chapter will help patients with tailbone pain to understand this approach. Note that while I advocate for using pelvic floor physical therapy (including manual medicine) for problems with muscles and tendons of the pelvic floor, this chapter is focusing specifically on manipulation of the coccyx.

## How Manipulation Is Done

Coccyx manipulation can be done by the health professional placing one or two fingers inside your anus and rectum, so these fingers are positioned in front of the tailbone. The health professional's thumb is then positioned behind the tailbone. This allows the clinician to grasp your tailbone in between his/her two fingers inside of you (that is the index finger and middle finger) and his/her thumb

> **Coccyx manipulation can be done by the health professional placing one or two fingers inside your anus and rectum.**

outside of you. The clinician can then push, pull, or rock your tailbone forward and backward. It is also possible to exert pressure onto the tailbone only externally (without inserting fingers into the anus and rectum), although this would only allow a limited direction of force to be applied.

The clinician who is manipulating your coccyx can perform the manipulation as a sudden, abrupt movement or as a more gentle, slow, sustained movement. The procedure may also include pressing on and stretching muscles, tendons and ligaments that attach to the tailbone.

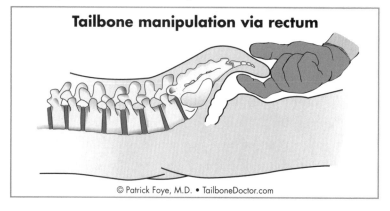

**Tailbone manipulation via rectum**

© Patrick Foye, M.D. • TailboneDoctor.com

Sometimes this is done as "manipulation under anesthesia." The anesthesia is used to make you unconscious (or less conscious) to spare you from feeling the pain of the manipulation and to relax the pelvic muscles that attach to your tailbone.

## Reasons for Manipulation

Coccyx manipulation may be done to improve the mobility of a tailbone that is "too stiff." Stiffness within the coccygeal joints may theoretically improve by causing movement of the bones at each side of each joint.

Coccyx manipulation may be done to attempt correction of a tailbone that is "out of alignment." This is sometimes called "adjustment." The idea is to attempt to push or pull the tailbone back into a more normal alignment.

Despite these potential rationales that might suggest the usefulness of coccyx manipulation, there are also reasons against undergoing manipulation.

## Reasons Against Manipulation

Although in theory the idea of manipulation may seem to have some merit, there are multiple reasons why it is not very successful for tailbone pain.

1. One of the most common reasons for tailbone pain is **unstable joints of the tailbone** (coccygeal dynamic instability). (See Chapter 6: *Unstable Tailbone Joints: Dynamic Instability.*) This means that for a large percentage of people with tailbone pain the coccygeal joints already have excessive looseness, laxity or mobility. Manipulation could cause further worsening of the unstable joints, thus making the underlying condition even more problematic and more difficult to treat.

2. Another common cause of tailbone pain is a **bone spur at the lower tip of the coccyx.** This additional bony extension (spur) is firmly attached to the lower tailbone. The only way to "manipulate" it away from the rest of the tailbone would be to forcefully fracture the spur to separate it. Highly undesirable.

3. A **fractured bone** needs time and rest for the fracture to heal. This is why fractures at other body sites are often stabilized within a cast or brace. Intentionally manipulating (mobilizing) the fractured bony pieces would be contraindicated (recommended against). Such stresses and movements at the fracture site could make the fracture unstable and could delay fracture healing.

   The combination of unstable joints, bone spurs, and fractures make up the *majority* of patients with tailbone pain. Since the paragraphs above explain why coccyx manipulation would be unlikely to help with each of these conditions (and could worsen them), manipulation may actually be contraindicated (inadvisable) in a *majority* of people with tailbone pain.

4. Even for patients who do have a **coccygeal bone that is out of alignment,** pushing or pulling it back into alignment will not necessarily get it to "stay" in that "properly aligned" position. In fact, for many patients with unstable joints of the tailbone, the coccyx bones go in and out of alignment multiple times throughout the day. For example, there may be normal alignment obtained just by standing up (which takes your seated body weight off of the tailbone). In that sense, the manipulation may do no more than what you are already doing by alternating between sitting and standing during the day, except that the manipulation may do this more forcefully.

5. Some patients experience **substantial exacerbation** (worsening) of their tailbone pain after the coccyx is manipulated. For patients who already have increased sensitivity and pain, undergoing a forceful manipulation can worsen the symptoms.

6. Manipulation clinicians often recommend that the procedure be repeated frequently, sometimes recommending a series of **dozens of manipulation sessions.** They sometimes even recommend continuing this even despite the initial sessions failing to provide relief.

7. If you are like many people, you may dislike the idea of the clinician's fingers being inserted into your anus and rectum, particularly on a frequently repeated basis.

## Who Performs Coccyx Manipulation?

Although theoretically anyone can perform coccyx manipulation (even patients themselves, or their spouses), the clinicians typically most skilled and experienced in this area include chiropractors, physical therapists (if they have special training in pelvic floor abnormalities), osteopathic physicians, and other musculoskeletal doctors.

## Effectiveness of Coccyx Manipulation

French research in 2001 concluded that coccyx manipulation gave a satisfactory outcome in only 25 percent of patients after six months, and even less satisfactory results after two years. This means that 75 percent of coccydynia patients fail to get a satisfactory outcome from manipulation.

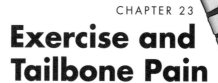

# CHAPTER 23

# Exercise and Tailbone Pain

## Emily's Story

Although Emily's job as a customer service representative was sedentary, outside of work she was physically very active and fit. Her favorite exercises included cycling and use of a rowing machine, activities that required sitting. When she developed tailbone pain that limited her from doing these activities, she began to feel frustrated, depressed, and out of shape. Emily's tailbone pain was treated with a local injection and occasional oral medications. Importantly, we also recommended modifications to her exercise program that allowed her to resume the activities she loved.

She started using padded cycling pants and a special bike seat to allow her to cycle again. She started varying her workout routine to include running, stair-climbing, and occasional swimming, so that her exercises did not always involve sitting. We advised her regarding which yoga exercises would aggravate her tailbone and which ones would not. Emily was able to resume an active and healthy lifestyle, accomplishing the fitness level that was so important to her overall sense of well-being.

If you have tailbone pain, you may wonder what exercises may help you versus hurt you. In this chapter you will discover exercises that may cause or exacerbate tailbone pain and other exercises that are safer and more helpful for you.

## Exercises That Cause or Exacerbate Tailbone Pain

Many exercises cause direct pressure on the tailbone. This pressure can cause or worsen tailbone pain. Some exercises result in an isolated, abrupt instance of trauma to the tailbone. Other exercises cause repetitive forces onto the tailbone, where the trauma is more gradual as it adds up from multiple small instances. Whether the traumatic forces on the tailbone are due to an isolated, sudden instance or due to repetitive trauma, injury and pain can result.

**Exercises can cause the start of coccyx pain in someone who previously had no tailbone symptoms.**

These exercises can cause the start of coccyx pain in someone who previously had no tailbone symptoms. Or, they may cause reappearance or worsening of tailbone pain in someone who already had a prior history of tailbone problems.

## Exercise Example: Sit Ups

To perform a traditional sit up, you typically start by lying flat on your back and then bend forward at the waist to come into a sitting position. Then you go backward again to the starting position. This is done repetitively to strengthen abdominal and other muscles. Each time that you come forward and each time that you go backward, you are putting your body weight onto your buttocks region, including your coccyx. The coccyx is part of the "fulcrum" upon which you are repetitively bending, or rocking, forward and backward. This can cause or worsen tailbone pain.

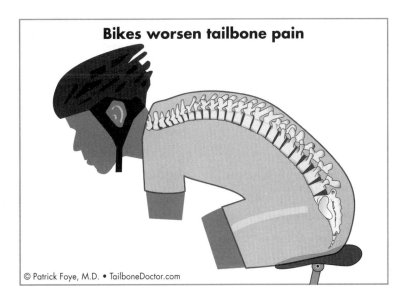

**Bikes worsen tailbone pain**

© Patrick Foye, M.D. • TailboneDoctor.com

## Cycling

Bicycle seats are often the most narrow seats we sit on. Your upper body weight (from the pelvis up) is forced down upon a narrow area. Then the repetitive cycling movement of each leg can cause the body weight to shift slightly from side to side while teetering on the tailbone at the midline. If you're cycling out on the street or off-road, there are bumps and potholes that add jarring forces onto the tailbone.

Aside from avoiding cycling altogether, there are some potential solutions. Many bicycle shops sell bike seats that have a cut-out for the tailbone. Also, wider bicycle seats will distribute the body weight across more of the buttocks and ischial bones (sit bones), which takes some of the pressure off of the tailbone.

Raising the height of the bike seat may help, by causing you to then bend, or flex, forward further at the waist. This forward flexion helps take pressure off the coccyx. The upper body weight shifts from the coccyx to the genital region and pudendal nerve region, which unfortunately can cause problems in those areas.

Padded cycling pants can provide cushioning for the tailbone. The padding over the coccyx area can absorb some of the shock and pressure.

It is possible to cycle without sitting. Some cyclists continue riding despite tailbone pain by riding (or doing spin class) while standing up on the foot pedals the entire time. By avoiding sitting on the bike seat, you can avoid causing pressure and exacerbation at your tailbone. But beware of causing problems in other body regions. Standing up will raise the height of your shoulders and arms, making it more difficult to reach the handlebars and potentially causing more of your upper body weight to be supported by your arms, putting them at risk for repetitive stress injuries.

## Rowing, Canoeing, Kayaking

Rowing exercise (whether paddling a canoe or kayak or using a rowing machine at the gym) puts direct pressure on the tailbone. While rowing, you typically tilt, or rock, your body weight forward and backward with each rowing stroke. This causes repetitive forces onto the tailbone. Meanwhile, the seat in the canoe or kayak is typically hard (wood or plastic, without padding) and unforgiving.

## Yoga

Yoga is a relatively safe form of exercise and meditation. However, there are some yoga poses that do place significant pressure directly onto the tailbone.

During "boat pose," you not only sit leaning backward but then also elevate your feet and legs. This combination of actions maximizes the pressure on your tailbone, since both the upper and lower body weight is then supported by your tailbone region.

"Lotus pose" involves sitting straight up, often with your legs crossed in front of you. Lotus pose places less pressure on the tailbone than boat pose does, but people tend to stay in lotus pose much longer, for example, while meditating. Prolonged time in lotus pose means prolonged pressure on the tailbone.

Some yoga positions are only problematic for the tailbone if you accidentally fall during the pose. Firefly pose requires using your arms to lift your body weight off the floor while your feet and legs are elevated off the floor. In firefly pose, the tailbone hovers above the floor. If balance or arm fatigue causes you to fall from this position, you will land directly on your tailbone region.

## Recreational Exercises or Activities

There are many other recreational activities that provide exercise but put the tailbone at risk for injury or pain. Some of these put direct pressure repetitively onto the tailbone. These include horseback riding, jet skiing, and going down waterslides.

Other recreational activities put pressure on the tailbone mainly only if you fall onto your tailbone during the activity. These activities include snowboarding, snow skiing, waterskiing, ice-skating, basketball, hockey, and martial arts.

## Exercises That Usually Do *NOT* Cause or Worsen Tailbone Pain

There are many exercises that can help your overall fitness with minimal risk to your tailbone. For most people, these exercises include walking, jogging, running, climbing stairs, using elliptical machines, swimming, and pretty much any other exercise you can think of that does not involve putting your body weight onto the tailbone.

Exercise has many benefits. So you should find the best activities that allow you to stay physically active. Exercise causes your body to release endorphins (chemicals that decrease pain). Exercise helps you to lose any excess body weight. Exercise causes an overall sense of well-being. The key of course is to find exercises that help you without worsening your tailbone pain or other conditions.

## Exercises with Physical Therapy

Exercise is a cornerstone of most physical therapy programs. Physical therapists can teach you exercises that help with many causes of low back pain and buttock pain. Exercises for pelvic floor pain are more challenging, but a growing number of physical therapists have expertise in this area. Exercises can help with muscular pain in the lower back, buttocks and pelvic floor. You may benefit greatly from finding a skilled physical therapist in your locality. There are also excellent books available on pelvic floor physical therapy.

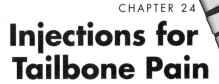

CHAPTER 24

# Injections for Tailbone Pain

## Sarah's Story

Sarah's local doctor had twice injected her tailbone blindly (without the image guidance of fluoroscopy) and without first making a diagnosis about what was causing Sarah's pain. The injections gave only minimal, temporary relief. So Sarah incorrectly assumed that this meant injections would not be a helpful treatment for her. But she traveled to our Tailbone Pain Center where we identified the specific tailbone joint that was causing her pain. Injecting that specific joint under the confirmation of fluoroscopic guidance provided excellent relief. All injections are *not* the same.

## Injections Compared with Medicines by Mouth

One problem with medications taken by mouth for tailbone pain is that the medications travel throughout your body, not just to the specific, focal site where you need them. This can put you at risk for side effects throughout your body, including bleeding stomach ulcers, constipation, liver impairment, kidney problems, heart attacks, strokes, and sedation (sleepiness and fuzzy thinking).

If you have a condition causing pain and inflammation throughout the entire body, it may make sense to accept the risks of taking a medication that travels through the entire body. But if you have a very focal, localized site of pain or inflammation (such as isolated tailbone pain), then it makes sense to deliver the medication focally just to that site. This is where injections play such a helpful role.

Since injections can deliver medication very specifically and focally to an exact site of injury or pain, it is extremely important that the treating physician first has looked for the specific cause of pain. You do not want to undergo a casual, somewhat randomly placed injection without first having a physician investigate the specific cause of pain. Otherwise, how would the doctor know whether an injection was needed or where best to place the injection?

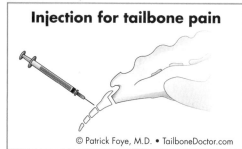

### Injection for tailbone pain

© Patrick Foye, M.D. • TailboneDoctor.com

In this chapter, you will discover the different types of injections that treat tailbone pain. You will learn the benefits and rationale for these treatments. You will also learn the difference between "blind" injections versus injections guided by fluoroscopy.

## Blind Injections versus Using Fluoroscopy

Tailbone injections are generally safe and effective at placing the medication at the proper location when done using image guidance. Fluoroscopy provides images that resemble an x-ray shown on a computer monitor. This allows the injecting physician to see your specific tailbone anatomy and compare this with the findings from your previous x-rays, MRI(s) or physical exam.

Unfortunately, many doctors still attempt "blind" coccyx injections, sticking a needle in the tailbone area and hoping for the best. In some cases they may get lucky and provide some relief. Alternatively, they may miss the target location. A blind injection at the wrong site is not only unhelpful, it can be harmful.

There is substantial variability in tailbone anatomy from one person to another. You may have three coccygeal bones, or four, or five. You may have wide joint spaces between all the bony segments, or have complete fusion of all of these coccygeal joints. Your tailbone may angle backward, or straight down, or forward. Fractures and dislocations further distort the anatomy, making blind injections even less reliable. As the lower tailbone commonly angles forward, it is a little deeper than can be confidently injected without image guidance. For all of these reasons, image guidance is considered superior to blind injections at the coccyx.

In modern times, fluoroscopy provides images to guide the physician to inject the ideal location. Older techniques included using CT scans during the injection, but that approach required substantial radiation exposure to the patient and a long injection time. Future approaches may include ultrasound guidance, but at the tailbone the standards for ultrasound guidance have not been established yet and would typically only show the most superficial outline of the bones closest to the skin. For now, fluoroscopy is the best choice for tailbone injections.

## Anti-inflammatory Steroid Injections

Inflammation is a common problem at sites of musculoskeletal pain, including the coccyx. Most people already know that inflammation is caused by arthritis, bone spurs, bone contusions and joint dislocations at other parts of the body, such as the shoulder, finger or foot. So it is no surprise that these same musculoskeletal conditions cause inflammation when they occur at the tailbone.

Inflammation is often excessive, resulting in more pain and tissue destruction. Anti-inflammatory medications taken by mouth, like ibuprofen, seek to decrease this inflammation and pain. But most of the dose taken by mouth goes throughout the body to sites distant from your tailbone. So the rationale for a local anti-inflammatory injection is to give the medication focally and locally, right where you need it.

The specific site for the steroid injection of course depends on the individual patient. There are multiple joints between the coccygeal bones, and often it is just one of these joints or bones that is involved in your pain, dislocation, excessive movement, or other injury. Or, perhaps there is a focal bone spur down at the lowest tip of the tailbone. Fluoroscopic guidance allows the physician to see the bones and joint spaces, so that the steroid injection can be injected at or around the optimal specific location.

Steroid injections often take approximately two days to two weeks to bring substantial relief. As with many injections, some patients may have increased soreness for the first few days, while waiting for the steroid to have its anti-inflammatory effect. Most common is for the relief from steroid injections to kick in a week or two after the injection, or occasionally a bit later. The relief is often substantial and dramatic.

## Ganglion Impar Sympathetic Nerve Blocks

The "sympathetic" nervous system is part of the human "fight or flight" response. Thousands of years ago, if a lion or tiger approached us then our bodies would kick into overdrive. Our heart rate and blood pressure would go up. Pupils of our eyes would widen to see more. More blood-flow would go to our muscles, to prepare us to respond. We would respond with "fight or flight," that is, either battling against the threat or running away from it! This response is hardwired into our nervous system. Sometimes these nerves can go into overdrive even when there is no real threat. Sometimes these overactive nerves (of the sympathetic nervous system) can become excessively sensitive to stimuli, including painful stimuli. When this happens, a touch or pressure that normally causes little or no pain now causes severe pain (out of proportion to the stimuli). This is called "sympathetically-maintained pain." (See Chapter 12: *Sympathetic Nervous System Pain at the Coccyx.*)

One treatment for sympathetically-maintained pain is to perform a sympathetic nerve block. A nerve block is when a local anesthetic is injected to bathe a nerve, which then becomes blocked (shut off). Local anesthetics include lidocaine (lignocaine, Xylocaine®), bupivacaine (Marcaine®), or in older days Novocain®. Although a pharmacist or chemist might say that the local anesthetics only work to block the nerve for a few hours, physicians and patients have known for many years that the treatment benefit can last for months or years, sometimes even giving permanent relief.

There are multiple comparisons used to explain this phenomenon where a local anesthetic (which chemically only lasts for a few hours) can produce relief that lasts for months, years or permanently. It is similar to having problems with your computer, where a few minutes of rebooting the computer results in the computer processing system getting back in order and functioning properly from that point forward.

The beneficial results are also compared to resetting a thermostat. You can "reset" a thermostat so that your air conditioning cools your home to a lower temperature. Similarly, anesthetic blocks of the sympathetic nervous system can "reset" nerves so that your baseline pain is at a lower level.

Ganglion Impar sympathetic nerve blocks should be done using image guidance (such as fluoroscopy) to help ensure that the medication is safely and effectively injected at the proper location.

Combination injections often include a ganglion Impar sympathetic nerve block (for the "nerve pain" of the hyperactive sympathetic nervous system) combined with a corticosteroid (anti-inflammatory) injection for the musculoskeletal pain and inflammation.

## Diagnostic Coccyx Injections (Test Injections)

A diagnostic injection (test injection) is when the physician injects local anesthetic to numb a specific site to see if this relieves your pain. This is helpful if the cause of pain is not completely clear. If injection at a very specific location relieves most or all of your pain, this shows that most or all of your pain is coming from that specific site or through those specific nerves.

> **Tailbone injections can provide medications locally at the specific site where you need them most.**

A test injection can also help in determining treatment options. For example, if you are considering nerve ablation to destroy the nerves carrying pain from the coccyx, a test injection can help show whether nerves at a specific site are carrying most of your coccyx pain. If numbing the nerves at one specific site relieves most or all of your pain, then that same site may be a good location for nerve ablation (destruction) to stop your pain more permanently.

Choosing the best target site for a test injection requires first carefully reviewing your symptoms, physical exam findings, and imaging results. These steps are crucial in helping determine the specific site where a test injection is most likely to be helpful.

The amount (liquid volume) of anesthetic injected for the test injection is intentionally kept very small. This is so the area of anesthetic effect (numbing) remains very focal and precise. The test injection usually involves injecting only a fraction of a teaspoon of fluid volume. This small volume helps to ensure that the resultant relief is due to blocking the nerves near the tip of the needle (rather than due to overflow of the liquid anesthetic to other regions).

As with most other tailbone injections, using image guidance (fluoroscopy) is often necessary to help in being as specific and accurate as possible with the precise location of the test injection.

## Nerve Ablation

If cushions, medications by mouth, coccyx steroid injections, and ganglion Impar sympathetic nerve blocks have all failed to give adequate relief of your tailbone pain, then coccygeal nerve ablation (nerve destruction) is often the best next step.

Local anesthetics merely block (shut off) nerves for a few hours (after which the nerve wakes back up, often at a lower, reset level of pain). Ablation is different because the nerves are not merely shut off for a few hours, but instead ablation intentionally destroys those nerves.

The goal of ablation is to provide long-lasting, perhaps even permanent, relief.

Even if your coccyx bone spur, or arthritis, or other musculo-skeletal condition persists, ablation can prevent the problematic site from sending pain signals to your brain. Even if your coccyx continues to have its musculoskeletal abnormality, if it is not causing you any pain or other problems then your quality of life improves.

Before any nerve ablation, it is important to assess your risk for underlying cancer or infection. You would not want ablation to merely mask the warning signs (pain) of an underlying destructive problem. This can be assessed by a careful physician obtaining a detailed history, physical exam, and review of imaging studies (x-rays and MRI or CT scans).

The precise location of the nerve ablation is crucial. The ideal site varies from patient to patient.

Deciding on the best specific location for nerve ablation depends on two main factors. First, the physician should understand exactly where the tailbone pain is coming from (such as one specific dislocating joint, or one specific bone spur at the lower tip of the coccyx). Second, the site of ablation should match the site that was used for a successful test injection. If a test injection (diagnostic injection) with local anesthetic at one specific location provided excellent short-term relief, then the ablation injection should target that same specific site.

## PRP (Platelet Rich Plasma) Injections

Platelet-rich plasma (PRP) injections are a growing area of medical research in the treatment of injured muscles, tendons, ligaments, and joints.

Plasma is the liquid component of our blood, in which blood cells and various chemicals are suspended. Using a centrifuge to spin your own blood sample, a physician can selectively draw out a portion of your blood containing plasma and a high concentration of platelets. This is platelet-rich plasma, or PRP. Your PRP sample also includes many of your biologically active chemicals that help promote healing.

PRP injections for tailbone pain may hold promise in the near future. PRP injections may promote healing of coccygeal ligaments and joints, which could be especially helpful for patients with unstable joints of the tailbone (coccygeal dynamic instability). Ongoing research is needed. Crucial for effectiveness would be first identifying the specific site of coccygeal joint hypermobility (by using sitting-versus-standing dynamic coccyx x-rays) or other musculoskeletal abnormalities of the coccyx, so that the injections can target the appropriate, specific site.

## Prolotherapy Injections

Prolotherapy is short for "proliferation therapy."

Prolotherapy involves injecting chemical irritants into a weakened tendon or ligament, or into a joint space. The theory is that the irritant will kick-start or stimulate your body to heal and repair the weakened tendon, ligament or joint. Often, a series of repeat injections are given.

The irritant injected is often one of the following: a highly concentrated sugar (hyperosmolar dextrose), glycerine, phenol, or extracts from cod liver oil (sodium morrhuate). Alternatively, sometimes rather than an irritant, the injection may instead include growth factors, or chemicals that stimulate growth factors.

Some published research has suggested that prolotherapy may help relieve coccyx pain. Further research is needed.

As with PRP injections, prolotherapy injections may be worth trying in patients who want to avoid surgery (coccygectomy) but have not obtained adequate relief from steroid injections and nerve blocks.


## Viscosupplementation Injections

The thick, gel-like liquid within a normal joint helps create smooth joint movement. When this joint fluid becomes less thick (less gel-like) in osteoarthritis, the joint can feel stiff and painful. The good news is that we can inject some gel-like liquid back into the joint, to decrease the pain and stiffness. Adding the viscous gel into the joint is like adding a few drops of oil to a rusty door hinge.

Since these injections provide a thick (*viscous*) fluid given as an extra *supplement* into the joint, the medical term for this is *viscosupplementation*. These injections contain a chemical called hyaluronic acid. Brand name examples include Hyalgan®, Supartz®, Euflexxa®, Synvisc®, and Orthovisc®.

Currently, viscosupplementation injections are used mainly for osteoarthritis only at the knee joint. But there may be a role for these injections at other joints in the body, including arthritic joints of the coccyx.

## Stem Cell Injections

Stem cell injections are a growing area of medical research, including treatment for many painful musculoskeletal conditions. This may be a future area of treatment research for tailbone pain.

## Cement Injection ... Beware

Coccygeal hypermobility (excessive movement at the joint spaces between coccygeal bones) is a very common cause of tailbone pain. (See Chapter 6: *Unstable Tailbone Joints: Dynamic Instability*) So, at first thought, it may seem reasonable to inject surgical cement into the loose coccygeal joints. A single such case has been reported once at a medical conference.

However, there are multiple problems with injecting cement at the coccyx. The normal coccyx typically has movement, but cement would cause zero movement at that cemented joint. Also, patients with excessive movement at the tailbone often go in and out of this dislocation as they alternate between sitting and standing throughout the day. Unfortunately, it's possible for the cement to fuse the tailbone in the wrong position (that is, cementing the tailbone fused in the dislocated position rather than in normal alignment). So cement injections can certainly make your tailbone condition worse (and I have inherited at least one patient where such worsening has happened).

## Benefits and Potential Risks of Various Injections

The desired goal, or benefit, of tailbone injections is to relieve your pain and suffering, and thus to improve your quality of life. In addition to decreased tailbone pain, other benefits include improved sitting tolerance (increased ability to sit for a prolonged time or increased ability to sit without using the coccyx cushion). When you can sit more comfortably and for a longer duration, you are more likely to be able to tolerate going out to a movie or a restaurant with friends or family. You are more likely to be able to sit for a business meeting at work or at your computer workstation. You are more likely to be able to sit for a long plane flight for a business or personal trip. Your life can improve in so many ways. Possibilities open up. Simple things that others take for granted are back within your reach.

Yet another benefit of tailbone injections is decreasing the amount of pain medications that you need to take by mouth. By helping you to decrease your pain medications, we can decrease the side effects from those medications.

All medical treatments have potential benefits and also potential risks. Even taking a single dose of an over-the-counter pain medication carries a risk. It may interact with other medicines that you're taking, or cause problems of the stomach, intestines, liver, or kidney. One goal of giving medication by injection is to decrease the widespread variety of side effects caused by medications taken by mouth. However, there are some potential side effects even with medications given by local injection.

Probably the most common side effect after injection is soreness at the site. Fortunately, compared with what you are familiar with from having your blood drawn for lab work, the needle that I use for tailbone injections is much thinner and much shorter. The needle is short because the tailbone is relatively close to the skin. The needle is wispy thin because tailbone injections require more subtle finesse rather than needing any brute force from a big needle. Still, the medications injected are liquids that can create some pressure from the fluid volume injected. Many patients will report increased pressure or soreness at the injection site for the first few days after the injection. Gradually the injected medication is absorbed into the local tissues and the pressure sensation quiets down, usually within a few days.

Any time you pierce the skin (even just for a simple vaccination or to draw a blood sample), there is a small risk of infection at the site. This risk is minimized by an experienced doctor using good, sterile technique while performing the injection. This risk is extremely low, probably less than one case out of every few thousand injections.

Some potential side effects depend on the specific type of injection performed or medication injected. For example, corticosteroids injected close to the skin can cause temporary paleness, or whitening, of the skin in that specific area. There can also be some loss of the fat cells that are located beneath the skin. This is one reason why fluoroscopic guidance is important for tailbone injections, to help avoid injecting into this fat layer.

While most of the injected steroids stay local at the injection site, a small amount may be absorbed into the body as a whole. This may cause restless sleep and other hormonal symptoms. In diabetic patients, the blood sugar levels may increase. These effects occur in only a small percentage of patients and usually resolve quickly.

Patients who have a history of allergic reaction to contrast, latex or medications should let their physicians know this, so that those specific items can be avoided.

Ablation injections tend to be the most painful during the initial days or even weeks after injection. During this time, the nerve fibers that carry pain from the tailbone are dying off and are "crying out their last gasps" before withering away. Reinnervation (nerves growing back again) can occur at the coccyx, causing coccygeal sensations to return. If the nerves start carrying pain signals from the coccyx again, then repeat ablation (months or years after the prior ablation) may help to again provide excellent relief.

## Repeat Injections

While any of the tailbone injections can give permanent, lifelong relief, sometimes the benefit may wear off months or years later. Or a new traumatic tailbone injury may cause the pain to return. If the injection was extremely helpful (such as giving 100 percent relief for many months or years) then it usually makes sense to repeat that same specific injection in hopes of again providing excellent relief.

Sometimes there is an unfortunate stigma against having repeated injections. The idea of repeating an injection that is beneficial is like repeating your regular dose of medication for blood pressure, or high cholesterol, or other medical conditions. If the treatment works well but is not permanent, then it is often worth repeating. Fortunately, tailbone injections do not need to be repeated as often as medications you take for other medical conditions.

If a given type of tailbone injection is *not* helpful, especially if it's unhelpful again on a repeat injection, then it usually makes sense to move on to a *different* type of injection or treatment.

## Summary Points on Injections

There are a variety of injections that help relieve tailbone pain. Tailbone injections can provide medications locally at the specific site where you need them most. It often makes sense to use a stepwise approach when deciding which injections to do. Repeat injections are often very helpful. Your treating physician should have the knowledge, experience and technical skills to provide you with the variety of available coccyx injections, and to be able to help guide you through the available options.

### Free Bonus for You

For your free printable list of injections for tailbone pain, where you can document which injections you have had and your response to those, go to: **TailboneDoctor.com/forms**

CHAPTER 25

# Coccygectomy: Surgical Removal of the Tailbone

## Hannah's Story

Hannah's tailbone pain was unfortunately in the minority of cases that fail to respond favorably to nonsurgical treatment. So she underwent coccygectomy (surgical removal of the tailbone). As per routine, she was not allowed to sit for several weeks after the operation, to allow the area to heal. She took time off from work and family responsibilities. Unfortunately, her surgery was complicated by infection at the surgical site, requiring a repeat surgery to remove infected tissue. By 12 months after surgery, Hannah's pain was significantly better than it had been before surgery. But she still was not totally pain free, and she required occasional medications and injections to manage her pain.

Coccygectomy is surgical amputation (removal) of the coccyx (tailbone).

It seems crazy that modern day health care would offer surgical amputation (removal) as the only surgical treatment for a painful body part. We would think it barbaric if the only proposed surgical treatment for thumb pain was to amputate your thumb. Yet the only surgery for coccyx pain is coccygectomy.

Some surgeons may callously and incorrectly advise their patients that the tailbone is a useless structure in humans so if it hurts just cut it out and everything will be perfectly fine. There are multiple incorrect assumptions in this line of thought. First, even though humans do not have tails, the tailbone is not useless. The tailbone serves as an anchoring point (attachment site) for many pelvic floor muscles, tendons and ligaments. Second, even when the entire painful tailbone is surgically removed, most patients still have some degree of persistent pain. Further, the recovery time after surgery is often considered six months to a year, so it is not a decision to be taken lightly.

> **Coccygectomy is a surgery with notable short-term and long-term risks.**

Still, coccygectomy can be medically necessary and helpful in the small percentage of properly selected cases where nonsurgical treatments have failed to provide adequate relief. I send for surgical consultation approximately one patient out of every 30 or 40 who I see at our Tailbone Pain Center. Also, coccygectomy may be absolutely necessary in the rare cases where the person has a cancer at the tailbone.

## Risks of Coccygectomy

Coccygectomy is a surgery with notable short-term and long-term risks.

## Infection

Short-term, during the initial weeks or months after surgery, coccygectomy carries a high risk of infection at the surgery site. This is because the coccygectomy site is so close to the anus. While you would fairly easily be able to keep clean a surgical site at your shoulder, wrist or knee, unfortunately there is no way to keep sterile the coccygectomy site. Stool and fecal bacteria can easily contaminate the surgical site.

Published research by Dr. Wood (at Harvard Medical School) documented that after coccygectomy as high as 35 percent of patients have postoperative complications including wound problems (infection or persistent drainage). Meanwhile, Dr. Doursounian's research team in Europe showed that 15 percent of coccygectomy patients required repeat surgery due to infection at the coccygectomy site. That means that more than approximately one out of every six patients requires a *repeat surgery* due to infection. This is an extremely high complication rate compared with most other elective surgeries.

Infection at the surgical site may involve only the skin (cellulitis) and superficial soft tissues. However, a more problematic infection can extend deeper, involving the bones (osteomyelitis) of the sacrum or any remaining segments of the coccyx. (See Chapter 14: *Bone Infection Causing Tailbone Pain*.)

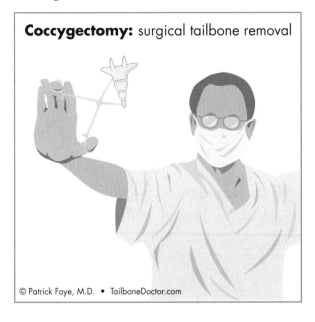

**Coccygectomy:** surgical tailbone removal

© Patrick Foye, M.D. • TailboneDoctor.com

## Persistent Pain

Some patients or surgeons may unrealistically expect that removing the tailbone is guaranteed to simultaneously remove all of the pain. But, unfortunately, *the majority of patients continue to have some persistent pain despite coccygectomy*. In fact, one British study by Eisenstein, et al., followed patients for an average of five years after coccygectomy and found that one-third of patients were unimproved.

Reasons for persistent pain despite coccygectomy include failure to remove the most symptomatic portion of the tailbone. Or scar tissue may form at the surgical site (perhaps causing compression or irritation of local nerves). Or perhaps the persistent pain has become "centralized," meaning that the pain source has eventually become located in the central nervous system and therefore can persist centrally even after the tailbone anatomy is removed. Or perhaps there is a persistent infection of the soft tissues or bone (osteomyelitis) at the surgical site.

Still, in the majority of properly selected patients undergoing surgical tailbone removal, there is significant decrease in overall pain, even if it is not resolved to zero. But it is important that the patient realize that complete relief only is obtained in less than 10 percent of patients undergoing the surgery.

Treatment for persistent pain after coccygectomy (post-coccygectomy pain) can include oral medications and local injections such as anti-inflammatory steroid injections, sympathetic nerve blocks, and nerve ablation.

## Pelvic Floor Prolapse

The pelvic floor is like a sling, or hammock, which holds up the pelvic organs, keeping them from falling toward the ground. Multiple muscles and ligaments of the pelvic floor attach to the tailbone. So when the tailbone is removed these structures lose one of their attachment sites. This can cause sagging (prolapse) of the pelvic floor.

When the pelvic floor sags (prolapses), the pelvic organs are no longer properly supported.

In women, the urinary bladder and uterus may start to sag (droop) or bulge downward toward the ground. This can cause not only pain but also urinary frequency and urinary incontinence (bladder "accidents").

In both men and women, sagging (prolapse) of the anus and rectum can cause fecal frequency, urgency, and incontinence (bowel "accidents").

Specialized physical therapy may help to strengthen the pelvic floor muscles. In some cases, surgery is needed to properly support these pelvic organs. Sometimes the uterus is surgically removed (hysterectomy) to lighten the weight that the pelvic organs put onto the pelvic floor.

As a complication of coccygectomy surgery, pelvic floor prolapse is probably seen in less than five percent of people who undergo the surgery. The risk is probably higher in women than in men, especially in those with any prior history of pelvic floor prolapse.

## Imaging Studies after Coccygectomy

When pain persists after coccygectomy, imaging studies should be done to investigate the cause of the persistent pain. I often inherit patients who have already undergone coccygectomy and have ongoing pain and yet unfortunately no imaging studies at all have been done after surgery to investigate the cause of the ongoing pain.

The imaging studies after coccygectomy can include x-rays, MRIs, and CT scans.

It is crucial that the imaging tests be ordered properly and performed properly, to include the specific site of pain.

After coccygectomy, a reasonable sequence would be to first obtain x-rays and then proceed to MRI, since MRI is better at showing any fluid collection, scar tissue, or infection within the bones or soft tissue. If bone infection is a concern, then additional advanced imaging studies could include a nuclear medicine bone scan (triple phase bone scan) or a labeled white blood cell scan.

## Outcomes of Coccygectomy

Despite the challenges discussed above, surgical removal of the coccyx is worth considering for the select patients who have not obtained adequate relief from nonsurgical treatment. In the majority of patients with focal tailbone pain, coccygectomy can significantly decrease the pain (but usually *some* pain continues). Also, if there is a cancer involving the coccyx, then surgically removing the coccyx may successfully remove the cancer.

## Summary

Coccygectomy (surgical amputation or removal of the tailbone) is typically reserved for the small number of cases where nonsurgical treatments fail to provide adequate relief. Or it is done to remove a cancer. Coccygectomy can have substantial short-term and long-term side effects, including infection, the need for repeat surgery, persistent pain, and pelvic floor prolapse. Still, coccygectomy provides significantly improved pain for most coccydynia (tailbone pain) patients. For persistent pain even after coccygectomy, oral medications and local injections can be helpful.

### Free Bonus for You

For your free printable checklist regarding evaluation and treatment for tailbone pain that continues despite coccygectomy, go to:
**TailboneDoctor.com/forms**

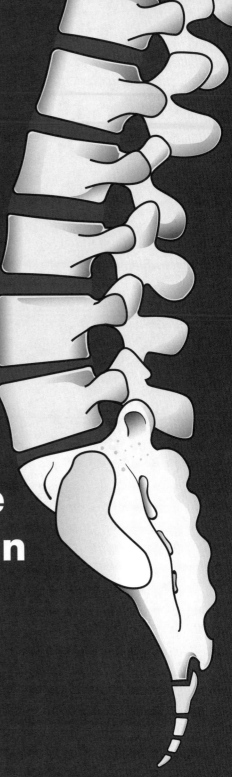

PART THREE

# Special Situations Regarding Tailbone Pain

## In This Section

**26** Working with Your Doctors......... 203

**27** Pregnancy, Childbirth and
Tailbone Pain ........................ 215

**28** Children with Tailbone Pain ....... 223

**29** Health Insurance for Tailbone Pain  227

**30** Legal Cases for Tailbone Injuries .. 239

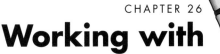

# CHAPTER 26

# Working with Your Doctors

## Donna's Story

When Donna's doctor seemed uninterested or unwilling to review with her the information she had found online regarding tailbone pain, she found another physician with a better bedside manner. She worked closely with the new physician to make sure that the correct tests were ordered, done, and carefully reviewed. She kept a folder with copies of reports from radiology imaging studies and injection procedure notes, along with the computer CDs containing the actual radiology images. When she eventually came for specialty consultation at our Tailbone Pain Center, her folder contained all the information needed to thoroughly review her prior workup and treatment. This formed a solid basis for recommending subsequent treatment options.

You can take an active, positive role in your own medical care for your tailbone pain.

The medical system is stacked against you if you have a relatively uncommon condition like tailbone pain. Some of your daunting challenges may include:

- finding a doctor who is knowledgeable about your condition,
- getting orders for the proper imaging tests,
- getting the radiology technician to perform the imaging studies properly for the tailbone,
- getting the radiologist to properly interpret the tailbone images,
- getting injections or other treatments from a physician skilled and experienced at performing them,
- finding a physical therapist with expertise in pelvic and coccyx problems, and
- getting your insurance company to understand and authorize the medical care that you need.

This chapter will help you discover active steps that you can take to effectively and diplomatically navigate the medical system.

## Finding a Physician

Finding a physician experienced at treating tailbone pain is often the best first step. Unfortunately, this can be challenging.

Try using Google or another search engine to search for terms such as "tailbone doctor" to see if there are any local physicians in your state or within traveling distance.

**Ask the doctor how many patients with tailbone pain he/she has treated in the past month.**

You can also search online at the United States National Library of Medicine's PubMed website. This site includes listings of medical publications from most major medical journals. Here, you can search for the term "coccydynia" to see if any of the medical authors are geographically close to you. The link for this is: *http://ncbi.nlm.nih.gov/pubmed/?term=coccydynia*

Call local doctors' offices, especially those specializing in musculoskeletal medicine, physical medicine and rehabilitation, sports medicine, or pain management. Specifically ask the receptionist if they treat "coccydynia" (the medical term for coccyx pain). If the receptionist has never heard of the term or sounds uncertain (or if you need to explain what that term means), then most likely the doctors in that practice are *not* routinely treating patients with tailbone pain.

Look at the medical practice website to see whether they mention tailbone pain. If they list dozens of other conditions but do not mention *the coccyx,* then clearly treating coccyx pain is not a significant part of their medical practice.

When you meet with a possible treating physician, ask the doctor how many patients with tailbone pain he/she has treated in the past month.

Beware of physicians who don't take your tailbone pain seriously. Many physicians dismiss and minimize patients' tailbone symptoms. They fail to recognize the substantial way that these symptoms compromise your quality of life. That insensitive and outdated approach disempowers patients. It removes hope. Many patients are told just to "live with it" or "grin and bear it."

Here are examples of *incorrect information and bad advice* that many doctors unfortunately tell patients:

- There are no good medical tests to assess or diagnose the causes of tailbone pain. (Wrong!)

- There are no good treatments for tailbone pain. (Wrong!)

- There's no treatment except surgical removal of the tailbone. (Wrong!)

- There is nothing wrong with your tailbone. (Really? Then why does the tailbone hurt so much, Doc?)

- The pain is "all in your head." (Really, Doc? Well, it's actually at the tailbone.)

- Nothing can be done to help you. (Wrong!)

All of these are blatantly wrong. Those doctors are giving bad advice. Those doctors are probably *ignorant* about the modern tests and treatments for tailbone pain. They simply don't know any better.

Worse yet, such incorrect medical "information" (actually, it's misinformation) disempowers patients from finding better answers, because patients are given the false impression that helpful answers are nowhere to be found.

Get a second opinion if you are not satisfied with the first physician you see. Just as you might not find a perfect fit with the first car that you test drive, you similarly might not find a perfect

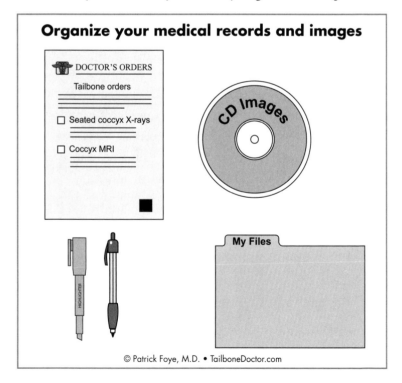

**Organize your medical records and images**

DOCTOR'S ORDERS

Tailbone orders

☐ Seated coccyx X-rays

☐ Coccyx MRI

CD Images

My Files

© Patrick Foye, M.D. • TailboneDoctor.com

fit with the first doctor you see for your tailbone pain. Do your best to see the most knowledgeable and experienced doctor you can find for your condition.

## Document Your Timeline

Document the timeline of your tailbone symptoms, tests and treatments. You can do this in a simple notebook, or on your smart phone, or in a computer document. There is great benefit to having even a simple, one-line, dated entry for each notable event, such as the onset of symptoms, tests (such as x-rays, MRIs), and any treatments that were provided. Memory and details will fade and merge over time. You don't need to write paragraphs, or even whole sentences. Just a date and a few words will often be enough to show what happened when.

## Helping Your Physical Exam

Your physician may not be experienced in doing a physical exam for tailbone pain, but you can help to at least partially make up for that inexperienced doctor.

Even before you go in for your doctor's visit, try to see if you can press over the painful area to reproduce your symptoms. To press (palpate) over the coccyx, feel for the area in the midline (in the "crack" between the right and left buttocks), just above and behind the anus and below the sacrum. If you feel a bony hardness there, that is the tailbone. If pressing that site reproduces your pain, consider marking the skin there with a black marker. Then, at your office visit with the doctor, ask your physician to look at the site you have marked. Ask the doctor to specifically press on that location and to confirm whether or not that is your tailbone. If your physician will not adequately look at the site and press there, find a different (better) physician.

If your doctor refers to your condition as "back pain" or "lumbosacral pain" despite the pain actually being down at the coccyx, diplomatically correct the doctor.

## Getting Proper Imaging Orders

The first step to getting proper radiology imaging studies of your tailbone is to get the orders from your treating physician. Some physicians incorrectly think it is useless to order the imaging studies because they incorrectly think that there are no treatments available regardless of what the imaging studies might show. But most physicians will at least order x-rays if you ask. Your doctor may even order an MRI.

If your doctor is ordering x-rays or an MRI, the next step is for you to make sure the images are ordered correctly. Every week at the Tailbone Pain Center I meet new patients whose previous x-rays, MRI, or CT scans failed to even include the coccyx. You can help avoid this happening to you with your imaging studies.

If your pain is at the coccyx, make sure that the radiology orders from your physician explicitly request images of the coccyx. Once your doctor has agreed to order imaging studies, diplomatically mention that you know that "lumbar" or "lumbosacral" images do not include the tailbone. Ask whether the orders will explicitly, specifically, and emphatically request images of the coccyx.

Look at the radiology orders that your doctor has written. Do the orders explicitly request images of the coccyx? If not, ask your doctor to modify the orders to specify this.

Ideally, if your tailbone pain is at its worst when you are sitting, then the side-view (lateral view) x-rays of your tailbone should be done while you are sitting, and compared with the side-view x-rays done while standing. Unfortunately, many radiology centers and radiology technicians will incorrectly tell you that there is no such thing as seated coccyx x-rays. They may look at you like you're crazy to even ask for such a thing. To have these extremely useful x-rays done properly may require traveling to a center that has more experience in treating tailbone pain.

## Radiology Technician Tips

Once you have the correct orders, the next challenge is getting the radiology technician to properly follow them. Because lumbosacral (low back) pain is probably 20,000 times more common than coccyx pain, the radiology technician may be on autopilot to perform lumbosacral imaging, even when your doctor has ordered coccyx or sacrococcygeal imaging.

You can and should explicitly tell the radiology technician that this is NOT lumbosacral pain, but instead is tailbone pain. Explicitly ask the radiology technician to enter tailbone pain as the reason for the test. This is important because the radiologist (physician) reading the images may never see the original orders from your treating physician. Instead the radiologist may only read the images based upon what the radiology technician has entered as the reason the studies were done. This is crazy but true.

Explicitly ask the radiology technician whether their technique will specifically include the tailbone. For MRI studies, bring a vitamin E capsule or ask the radiology technician if there is another marker that can be taped to the skin over the site of pain, to ensure that the painful area is included.

Some radiology centers have digital images that will be visible on the computer screen even while you are still in the exam room. Some radiology technicians may allow you to look at the images before you leave, and you can ask them to point out your tailbone to you. Although the technician is probably not officially credentialed or allowed to give you a diagnostic interpretation of the images, sometimes he/she may give you an unofficial impression, or at least be able to show you that the tailbone is included in the images.

## Imaging Results

Every time you have radiology imaging studies done, you should make sure to get a copy of the official, typed, radiology report. You should be able to get this directly from the radiology center where you had the study performed. If not, then be sure to obtain a copy of the report from the office of the doctor that ordered the test.

When you receive a copy of the radiology report, review it with a yellow highlighter. Highlight your name (to confirm that the report is really about you!), the study date, and the type of study (x-ray versus MRI versus CT scan). All of this will make this document very easy to find and refer back to in the future.

Next, read the radiology report and highlight every place where you see the words coccyx, coccygeal, or tailbone. If nowhere within the radiology report it ever explicitly mentions the tailbone (despite tailbone pain being the reason that the study was done), then you or the ordering physician can request that the radiologist provide an official, typed addendum to the report, addressing the tailbone.

If there are terms within your imaging report that you do not understand, look them up on Google or another Internet search engine, or make a note for yourself to ask your physician about these at your next follow-up visit.

Review the imaging report with your physician. Have your doctor explain the findings. Have your doctor especially review what it explicitly says about the tailbone, as well as any abnormalities in other areas.

If the radiologist recommended any follow-up studies (such as diagnostic ultrasound for abnormal findings at the uterus or ovaries), then have your doctor give you the orders to have those follow-up studies done. Share the radiology report with your other treating physicians, especially if their expertise overlaps with any positive findings (such as your gynecologist for findings in the female reproductive organs, or your gastroenterologist for findings in the colon or rectum).

## Getting the Actual Images

In addition to obtaining and reviewing the typed, paper report, you should also obtain and review the actual images. These will be available from the radiology center, either on films or on a computer CD.

Images on film can be expensive, and they are large, heavy, and awkward to carry or mail. Images on computer CD are often free and the CD is small enough to easily fit in your purse or file folder, or into a padded mailing envelope. If you know how to make a copy of the CD from your home computer, you can keep one copy for yourself while giving other copies to your treating physicians. Some radiology centers will mail the computer CD directly to the ordering physician, while others will give the CD directly to you, and others may do both. Always ask, because some radiology centers will not share the actual images at all unless it is explicitly requested.

## Reviewing the Actual Images

Once you have your actual images (on CD or films), ideally you should have a follow-up visit with the ordering physician to review both the typed (paper) radiology report and the actual images.

Ask your doctor to point to your tailbone on the radiology images. My medical students and resident physicians call this "Dr. Foye's finger-pointing test" for coccyx imaging. To me this seems so basic that it should hardly need mentioning, but I give this tip to people suffering with tailbone pain around the world, and I very frequently hear back that the results were profoundly revealing.

You may be amazed to find that your doctor is unable to point out your tailbone on the imaging studies, either because he/she is inexperienced at reviewing tailbone images, or perhaps because the images failed to include the tailbone at all. If the images failed to include the coccyx, consider having the radiology center complete the study (including the coccyx) at no additional charge.

Or, you and your doctor may indeed be able to see the coccyx but be amazed that you have a blatant coccyx abnormality that the radiologist failed to mention. If that happens, you or your doctor can call the radiology center and ask for a formal addendum to the radiology report.

If your treating physician does not want to take the time to look at your coccyx images, consider finding a different physician.

## Record-Keeping

For any medical condition that you or your family member has, I recommend starting a simple folder in which you keep copies of imaging reports, consultation notes, etc. Also keep a copy of your timeline (a simple list of dates and what test or procedure was done on each of those dates).

Ask your doctor's office for a copy of your office visit medical notes, explaining that it will help you to be able to review and make sure you understood and remembered everything the doctor went over. Those notes are also important if you see another medical specialist, who will want to review those previous records. When sharing medical notes and radiology reports with a new physician, be sure to keep a set of copies for yourself.

Use your yellow highlighter to highlight the main points of a given office visit note. Start by highlighting your name (to make sure the note is about you!) and the date. Then highlight important parts that explain any new diagnosis that was made, or any "action items," such as any plans for additional testing, treatments or consultations.

## General Questions for Your Doctor

Especially if your physician is not experienced with treating tailbone pain, there are some important questions that you can diplomatically ask to help move your medical care forward. Some examples are listed below.

- "Have you had previous patients with similar symptoms? If so, what tests or treatments or specialists were helpful?"

- "What type of imaging study or other test would I get if this were pain in my thumb? Can I get a tailbone-version of that test for my coccyx?"

- "Is there any chance that this pain could be coming from other pelvic organs, such as the colon, the uterus or ovaries (in women) or the prostate (in men)?"

- "Is there any chance this pain could be caused by cancer?"

- "If this were affecting you or your family member, what testing would you do? Who would you go to for treatment?"

## Insurance Issues

You will probably need to work closely with your doctor to help your insurance company understand your medical needs and authorize the necessary testing and treatment. It may be helpful for you to contact your insurance company directly, to express the human side of your pain, suffering, and medical needs. This book includes an entire chapter about navigating the medical insurance system for patients with tailbone pain. (See Chapter 29: *Health Insurance for Tailbone Pain*.)

### Free Bonus for You

For your free printable checklist to help you track your tests and treatments for tailbone pain, go to: **TailboneDoctor.com/forms**

# CHAPTER 27

# Pregnancy, Childbirth and Tailbone Pain

## Brittany's Story

Brittany was excited about the birth of her first child. She imagined blissfully bonding with her baby. But her idealized expectations of her first months of motherhood were shattered by the coccyx dislocation that occurred during labor and delivery. Brittany could not sit up to hold and breastfeed her newborn son. She avoided taking pain medications due to the risks that these chemicals would be transmitted to her baby through her breast milk. But without pain medications she was in daily agony. What was supposed to be the happiest time of her life had turned into a nightmare. She cried and wondered, "How can this be happening to me?"

## Pregnancy versus Childbirth

This chapter addresses tailbone issues related to pregnancy separately from those related to childbirth (going into labor and delivering the baby). This separation is because pregnancy and childbirth are two distinctly different events with distinctly different effects on the tailbone.

## Pregnancy Causing Coccyx Pain

During pregnancy, there are substantial changes in the anatomical and mechanical forces within the mother's body. Pregnant women typically gain a substantial amount of body weight. Many have decreased levels of overall energy, especially later in the pregnancy. These factors may result in the pregnant woman becoming more sedentary, with more time spent sitting. Sitting puts a portion of the person's body weight directly onto the coccyx. Further, the woman's increased abdominal weight due to the pregnancy may have her sitting posture change such that she may often sit leaning partly backward, which puts even

**The baby's head and body may forcefully push the tailbone out-of-the-way, causing tailbone injury.**

further weight and pressure upon the tailbone. Women who may have had a pre-existing, underlying tailbone condition that was not previously causing any symptoms may now become symptomatic. For example, a woman may have years of laxity (looseness) of the joints between the coccygeal bones, or a bone spur (extra bone at the lower coccyx, causing a pointy tip that faces backward and pinches the skin when sitting leaning back). But these conditions may not have previously caused any pain or other symptoms until the pregnancy caused the additional physical, mechanical stresses onto the tailbone (due to increased weight, increased sitting and increased leaning backward while sitting).

In other cases, a woman may have previously experienced a tailbone injury or other painful coccyx condition, but that condition and its symptoms may have completely resolved only to return during the current pregnancy (again, due to the additional mechanical stresses as noted above).

Further, during the later weeks of pregnancy a woman's body creates increased levels of certain hormones that cause the ligaments within the pelvis to become more loose. Overall, this is very helpful in creating increased flexibility of the bony pelvis to prepare for and allow the baby to pass through the pelvic birth canal. However, in some patients this increased laxity may be excessive, causing ligaments at the coccyx to become too loose (lax). These excessively lax ligaments may cause the coccygeal joints to become unstable (unable to maintain normal alignment of the coccygeal bones). So, some women who have never previously had any tailbone pain or underlying tailbone condition may have new (first-time) onset of tailbone pain during pregnancy.

Now that we have addressed tailbone pain related to the pregnancy itself, we will move on to discussing the tailbone problems associated with actually giving birth.

## Childbirth (Labor and Delivery) Causing Coccyx Pain

During later stages of pregnancy, women create increased levels of a hormone that causes looseness (laxity) of ligaments within the pelvis. Typically, this laxity peaks around the time of childbirth, when the woman goes into labor and delivers the baby. This is a normal and helpful process, which helps allow the baby to be born through the pelvic birth canal. However, this increased looseness of the coccygeal joints may put the mother at increased risk for injury, since the joints have lost some of their normal, protective ligamentous support.

Next, when the baby moves from the mother's abdomen down into the pelvis and through the birth canal, this places dramatically increased stresses upon the pelvis. The pelvic bones, ligaments, muscles, and tendons all are placed under these increased mechanical forces and stresses. The tailbone is not spared from these stresses.

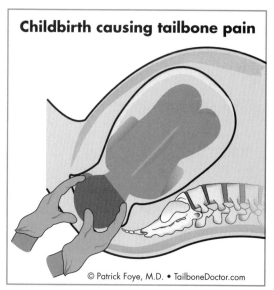

© Patrick Foye, M.D. • TailboneDoctor.com

These increased forces on the tailbone can cause tailbone fractures, dislocations, and other injuries. While the mother is pushing to deliver the baby, the mother and the medical birth team may actually hear a cracking sound as the tailbone is fractured.

In some women, the angle of the tailbone is flexed too far forward, where it unfortunately causes an obstruction of the birth canal. In these cases, when the baby starts passing through the birth canal the baby's head and body may forcefully push the tailbone out-of-the-way, causing tailbone injury.

Aside from the *internal* mechanical forces placed upon the tailbone from within the pelvis, there are also *external* forces that can cause problems. During childbirth, many women in Western societies are positioned sitting leaning backward onto a reclining exam table or hospital bed. Sitting leaning backward tends to be the worst possible position for tailbone pain.

A mother with a pre-existing tailbone condition (such as a bone spur that previously was not even causing any symptoms) may become symptomatic after hours of sitting leaning backward during childbirth.

In summary, there are both internal and external mechanical forces acting upon a woman's tailbone when she is giving birth.

## Coccyx Pain and Subsequent Pregnancy

Many women with current or previous coccyx pain are concerned about whether subsequent pregnancies will cause their pain to worsen or to return. This is a valid concern, since we know that coccyx pain can indeed be worsened both by pregnancy and by giving birth.

## Timing Related to Future Pregnancy

One important approach for a woman with coccyx pain is to treat the condition as thoroughly as possible BEFORE a subsequent pregnancy. This is important because many of the treatments will no longer be available to a woman while she is pregnant. For example, pregnant women are often advised to avoid using nonsteroidal anti-inflammatory drugs (NSAIDs) such as ibuprofen. Pregnant women should generally avoid getting x-rays or CT scans of the pelvic region, due to harmful radiation exposure to the developing fetus. Similarly, pregnant women should generally avoid injections at the tailbone or other pelvic regions during the pregnancy.

Thus, pregnant women are limited from some of the standard testing and treatment for tailbone pain. This makes it important for women to optimize their tailbone testing and treatment *before* any subsequent pregnancy.

## Vaginal Birth versus Cesarean Section (C-Section)

Pregnant women who have a history of previous or current tailbone symptoms should tell this to their medical birth team (obstetrician or midwife). Ideally, this conversation should take place well in advance of labor and delivery, so that the expectant mother and her team can have time to consider and plan for the delivery in advance.

I have seen many women with tailbone pain who go on to deliver vaginally without difficulty. Unfortunately, many other women who have attempted to do so have suffered a significant worsening of their pain. So, there is no single answer or approach that is best for every individual patient.

Some of this may depend upon factors such as the specific anatomic location of the tailbone in an individual patient. For example, a tailbone that is in a position of abrupt forward flexion (angled forward into the pelvis) may cause obstruction of the birth canal, raising the reasonable consideration for a delivery by cesarean section (instead of through the obstructed birth canal).

Alternatively, a woman with a bone spur projecting backward from the lower tip of the coccyx would have no obstruction of the birth canal and might be more capable of delivering the baby vaginally. Instead of cesarean section, perhaps this woman just needs better use of padding or cushioning so that she is not leaning backward onto the bone spur. Or she may need to change her position so that she does not spend labor and delivery leaning backward on a medical bed or table. Instead, she and her birth team may wish to consider having her deliver the baby in a squatting position.

## Already Pregnant and in Pain

If a woman is already pregnant and already experiencing tailbone pain, this is a challenging situation. The pregnant woman will typically spend more time sitting and sitting leaning back, which tends to worsen tailbone pain. Also, the woman and her birth team need to discuss and plan for the eventual childbirth, including considering vaginal delivery versus C-section.

Plans should also be made for evaluating and treating the tailbone pain after the baby is delivered. Sadly, the otherwise joyous occasion of a new baby can instead be a time of pain and suffering for a mother whose tailbone pain is not adequately addressed. So, even though there are many limitations to the testing and treatment available during the pregnancy, plans should be made to move forward with such medical care once the pregnancy is over. Parents' time and energy after delivery are understandably focused on the newborn, so having the mother's tailbone treatment plan in place before that can be extremely helpful. Also, having a plan in place can provide some level of reassurance to the pregnant woman who is suffering with tailbone pain.

## Breastfeeding

Breastfeeding (nursing) provides many advantages to the newborn in both nutrition and immune protection from certain infections. Breastfeeding also provides a bonding experience for the mother and her baby. But unfortunately, this experience can be dramatically compromised if the mother is suffering with tailbone pain while breastfeeding.

Tailbone pain is usually worse while sitting, and especially sitting leaning partway back. Yet this is a common position for women to be in while breastfeeding.

Alternative approaches include breastfeeding while side-lying (lying down instead of sitting). If breastfeeding needs to be done while sitting, then the mother should use a cushion with a cut-out in the tailbone region, to take the pressure off of her coccyx. (See Chapter 20: *Cushions for Tailbone Pain.*) Aside from the typical cushions for tailbone pain, many new mothers have discovered that it can be helpful to sit on a "Boppy." A Boppy® is a U-shaped cushion typically worn around the mother's abdomen to help her hold the baby during breastfeeding. Sitting on this Boppy with the "opening" of the U in the back (under the tailbone) can decrease the pressure placed upon the tailbone during sitting.

Also worth mentioning is that some medications that the mother may take to relieve pain may find their way into the breast milk. For example, opioid (narcotic) painkillers (such as oxycodone) can be very effective at relieving pain, but may be transmitted to the child in the mother's breast milk. A newborn receiving breast milk containing opioid painkillers may have problems such as increased sleepiness and constipation.

### Free Bonus for You

For your free printable checklist describing how to work with your gynecologist or midwife to minimize your tailbone pain during pregnancy and childbirth, go to: **TailboneDoctor.com/forms**

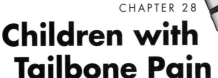

# CHAPTER 28

# Children with Tailbone Pain

## Isabella's Story

At 14-years-old, Isabella was a happy high school freshman until she slipped and fell on the wet tile floor at practice for the school's swimming team. She suffered from tailbone pain that persisted for many months. Her pediatrician incorrectly told her parents that there is no treatment available for tailbone pain and even suggested that maybe Isabella was just making up her ongoing symptoms. But that didn't make sense to her parents—they knew enough to believe in their child's reports of pain. They brought her to the Tailbone Pain Center, where she received an accurate diagnosis and helpful treatment.

As a parent myself of a child with multiple medical issues and surgeries, my heart goes out to children and their parents when I evaluate a child with tailbone pain. I am profoundly grateful to clinicians who made a positive difference for my own child's conditions. I strive to provide helpful care to those I treat for tailbone pain.

Tailbone pain in children is similar in many ways to tailbone pain in adults, but there are a few important differences. There are additional challenges in treating tailbone pain in children.

## Flexibility of Youth

One of the most common causes of tailbone pain is unstable joints of the tailbone (coccygeal dynamic instability), which is excessive laxity (looseness) at the coccygeal joints. This increased laxity of the joints unfortunately allows for excessive movement at those joints and bones when a person is weight-bearing at the coccyx while sitting.

> **There are additional challenges in treating tailbone pain in children.**

A certain amount of joint laxity is normal, but when it is excessive it is problematic. (See Chapter 6: *Unstable Tailbone Joints: Dynamic Instability*.)

Children, as a baseline, already have significantly more joint flexibility and laxity than adults do. So children may have a higher risk of having unstable joints of the tailbone.

The difficulty with diagnosing coccygeal dynamic instability in children is that the diagnostic criteria are based upon coccyx movement in adults, not children.

"Normal values" are established by looking at x-rays showing how much movement the tailbone has while sitting leaning backward, as compared with its position while

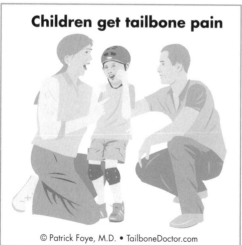

**Children get tailbone pain**

© Patrick Foye, M.D. • TailboneDoctor.com

standing. To establish how much movement is normal, these studies were done on people with no history of tailbone injury and no symptoms of tailbone pain.

These normal values (showing how much the coccyx moves while sitting) have been established for adults, but not for children. So, we end up using the normal-versus-abnormal cut off values that are known for adults, and we apply these to children. We know that doing so is not perfect, but this is the best data we have at this time.

## Avoid CT Scans

One concern for children with tailbone pain or other sites of pelvic pain is that CT scans can deliver a substantial amount of radiation to the child's reproductive organs.

I would not be so dogmatic to say that pelvic CT scans should *never* be done in children. But I would say that other imaging options should usually be considered first. For example, an MRI provides extensive anatomic detail without any of the radiation that CT scans impose.

X-rays can also deliver radiation, but typically this is far less than with CT scans. In particular, tailbone x-rays can be done using a "coned-down" view, which focuses the x-rays on the area of concern (the coccyx) while minimizing the radiation exposure to all other areas.

## Gym Restrictions

Physical education classes are often a required component of a child's school curriculum. But for the child with tailbone pain, certain physical activities need to be avoided, to minimize the chance of a painful exacerbation.

The treating physician can provide the child with a medical excuse note, indicating that the child should not perform gym activities that put direct pressure on the tailbone. These activities include avoiding sit-ups (and abdominal crunches), cycling, rowing, and a few yoga poses (such as boat pose).

## Classroom Accommodations

A child with tailbone pain may be unable to sit for the entire duration of multiple hours of class throughout the school day. As an accommodation, students should be allowed to use their tailbone cushion at school (although, admittedly, some teenagers would rather suffer the pain than carry a cushion from class to class). Students can also be provided with a medical note allowing them to stand intermittently throughout the school day. The student can stand at the back or side of the classroom. This should not be disruptive, so most reasonable teachers and school administrators will honor such a note from the treating physician.

## Treatments

In general, treatments for tailbone pain are similar in children and adults. For further details on treatment of tailbone pain, please see Chapters 18 through 25.

### Free Bonus for You

For your free printable template showing typical school gym restrictions for children with tailbone pain, go to: **TailboneDoctor.com/forms**

# CHAPTER 29

# Health Insurance for Tailbone Pain

## Matthew's Story

Matthew had assumed that his health insurance plan would efficiently cover his medical care if he ever became sick or injured. But when he developed tailbone pain he found that his insurance company repeatedly denied coverage for the tests and treatments that he needed. They were inappropriately making decisions based on criteria intended for patients with lower back (lumbar) pain rather than tailbone pain. Next, an insurance company representative even claimed that the coccyx was not part of the spine and therefore did not qualify for spine-related care. The patient and his physician had an uphill battle appealing the denials and obtaining coverage for his tests and treatments.

Health insurance in the United States has obstacles that are specifically problematic for people with tailbone pain. This chapter will help you navigate through, around and beyond those obstacles.

## Finding an Experienced Physician

Often, your first obstacle is finding a medical doctor experienced at treating tailbone pain. Your insurance company's long list of "in-network" providers is useless if none of them have adequate experience, training, or expertise treating tailbone pain.

## In-Network versus Out-of-Network

Insurance companies often have a list of doctors who are "in-network" with their insurance plans. This means that the doctor's office has signed a contract with your insurance company, typically agreeing to accept lower, discounted payments from your insurance company for the physician's services.

Meanwhile, the same doctor's office will be "out-of-network" with many other insurance plans. The reason for being out-of-network might be that the insurance company is requesting such deep discounts that the medical office finds the insurance company's fee schedule unacceptably low. Or, even more commonly, it is simply not practical for any one doctor's office to complete all the substantial paperwork, applications, and legal contract review with each and every insurance plan in the country, or even in one geographic region. There are just too many insurance plans to keep up with.

If you find a medical doctor experienced in treating tailbone pain who is in-network with your insurance plan, that is terrific. But often for specialized care like this you will need to look out-of-network.

## Out-of-Network Benefits

Many insurance plans do still provide insurance coverage for you even if you decide to see physicians outside of their network. Often they will cover this using your "out-of-network benefits." Although this may involve higher "out-of-pocket" expenses than you would pay for an in-network physician, this may be worthwhile and necessary to find the care and expertise that you need and deserve.

Sometimes even if your insurance plan does not have any out-of-network benefits, your insurance company may still decide to provide insurance coverage for you to see an out-of-network specialist. You may need to demonstrate to them that the type of medical subspecialty care that you require is not available from any in-network provider. For example, at our Tailbone Pain Center there are some specialized medical services that usually cannot be readily obtained through your local doctors. Based on this, you may be able to successfully appeal to your insurance company to cover your medical care with an out-of-network physician, even if your policy says that you do not have any out-of-network benefits.

## Referral

Your insurance company may require that you have a referral from your primary care physician in order to see a specialist.

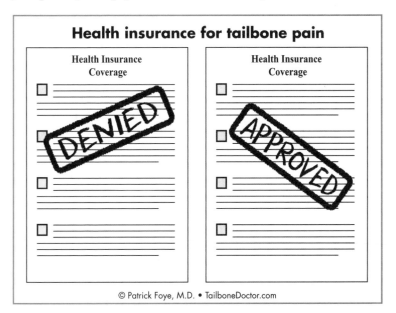

### Health insurance for tailbone pain

Health Insurance Coverage

Health Insurance Coverage

© Patrick Foye, M.D. • TailboneDoctor.com

## Keep a Notebook

Being organized is well worth the initial time and effort when navigating your way through the health insurance system.

You should keep a notebook or folder where you document any communications you have with your insurance company. Each time you call them, document the date, the name of the person you spoke with, any reference number for the call, and a summary of any information, recommendations, or decisions that they gave you. This will be extremely helpful for later reference if your insurance company fails to follow through on something they promised you. This information also helps you generate a "to-do list" of any actions you need to take to move your care forward.

> **You and your treating physician need to be extremely explicit and thorough in explaining to your insurance company exactly what type of test or treatment is needed.**

## Pre-Authorizations

Some insurance plans require pre-authorization (pre-certification) before you can undergo medical tests (such as MRI), physical therapy, injections, or other treatments. This means that the insurance company must approve the test or treatment before the service is provided, not afterward. You or your healthcare provider should check with your insurance company in advance of doing these services, to find out whether pre-authorization is needed. If pre-authorization is required, your doctor's office may need to call the insurance company by phone and answer questions about your medical details. Your doctor's office may also need to fax your medical records to the insurance company for its review. This can require hours of phone calls and days (occasionally weeks) of waiting for an insurance company to respond.

## Criteria for Pre-Authorizations

Your insurance company may have formal criteria upon which it bases the decision to approve or deny requests for coverage of your medical care. Whenever possible, you should absolutely try to obtain a copy of the criteria used for the medical service you are seeking. Never trust that the insurance company employee is giving you the correct information by phone. You need to see the criteria yourself, in writing, to know if it is actually the correct criteria for your condition and whether the employee is interpreting and applying the criteria appropriately. Similarly, if you receive a letter denying authorization, you need to follow up by requesting a written copy of the policy or criteria upon which the denial was based.

Pre-authorization criteria often look at factors such as how long your pain or other symptoms have been present. The criteria often seek to encourage the use of the least expensive tests or treatments first. For example, in requesting pre-authorization for a tailbone injection, it is important to inform your doctor and insurance company if you have already tried many weeks or months of ibuprofen and other pain medications, a coccyx cushion, or other methods to relieve pain.

Because tailbone pain is relatively uncommon, many insurance companies do not have explicit criteria regarding the tests or treatments specifically for tailbone pain. Frequently, insurance companies incorrectly apply criteria for lumbar pain (low back pain at about the level of the belt line) even though what you have is tailbone pain, totally different from the lumbar region. By reading the criteria yourself (perhaps with the help of your treating physician) you will be able to spot the errors. Then, you and your physician can both diplomatically but firmly inform your insurance company that it has used the criteria inappropriately and that those criteria do not apply to this specific anatomic site at the tailbone.

## CPT Codes

In the United States, different medical tests and treatments are assigned specific numbers for medical billing. These numbers (codes) are called CPT (Current Procedural Terminology) codes.

Almost every medical test or treatment you can imagine has been assigned a unique CPT code. One problem for patients with tailbone pain is that some tests and treatments specifically at the tailbone do not have any such CPT code.

For example, there is no CPT code that explicitly covers MRI of the tailbone (coccyx). There are different CPT codes for MRI of every other region of the vertebral spine (cervical, thoracic and lumbosacral), but none for the coccyx. A lumbosacral MRI does not include images low down enough to show the coccyx. There is a CPT code for "pelvic" MRI, but the pelvic MRI focuses mainly on pelvic organs (urinary bladder, uterus, ovaries, etc.) and does not include the midline sagittal images needed to best show the coccyx. A standard pelvic MRI does not focus far enough back in the pelvis to give optimal views of the coccyx.

Your physician has two options, and both of them are bad. Neither the lumbar MRI nor the pelvic MRI optimally shows your tailbone. Requesting pre-authorization for the CPT code for a lumbar (or lumbosacral) MRI may result in denial by the insurance company, because your pain down at the tailbone will not fulfill the criteria to have an MRI done up at the lumbar region. Similarly, requesting pre-authorization for the pelvic MRI CPT code may result in denial by the insurance company, because you do not have symptoms in the pelvic organs that the pelvic MRI would focus on.

All of this means that you and your treating physician need to be extremely explicit and thorough in explaining to your insurance company exactly what type of test or treatment is needed, along with how the requested services are similar yet distinctly different from the available CPT codes.

With time, effort and persistence these obstacles can usually be overcome. But they are challenges above and beyond those faced by other patients whose medical conditions are much more common than tailbone pain.

## Appealing Denials

If your insurance company denies authorization for a test or treatment, you can usually appeal the denial. There is a formal process for this. Usually the appeal must be done in writing and must be done before a specified deadline. Usually the appeal will be done by the treating physician's office. But as the patient, you can additionally call your insurance company directly to help them understand the human side of your pain and suffering.

You or your treating doctor should try to obtain a copy of the specific criteria or reason that the insurance company used to deny a test or treatment, since that information may help form the basis of your appeal.

## Your Human Resources or Benefits Office

Health insurance is commonly provided through your employer (or your spouse's employer). If you are having substantial difficulties with your insurance company, you may be able to find help and support through your employer's human resources office or benefits office. Insurance companies realize that unresolved complaints that they receive through your employer may cause the insurance company to lose future business with your employer. If you have a helpful ally at your employer's benefits office, this can be very useful when you are requesting pre-authorizations, or appealing a denial, or requesting to see an out-of-network physician. Your ally can contact the insurance company on your behalf and encourage authorization of the necessary medical care.

## "Experimental" Treatment

Sometimes an insurance company will deny coverage for a treatment because they label it as "experimental." This is a subjective term, often based on just the opinion of whoever is reviewing your medical case.

Frequently, insurance companies will label treatments as "experimental" (and therefore deny payment for those treatments) even though the treatment is well established within the medical community and within medical publications. This incorrect labeling of a treatment as experimental inappropriately denies the patient their medical care and coverage. The denial may be caused by the insurance company's reviewer being ignorant or inexperienced in the area of tailbone pain.

Other times, the treatment may indeed be experimental, meaning that its effectiveness has not yet been established by published medical research. You may decide to proceed anyway if the treatment seems to be worth trying, even if your insurance company will not pay for the costs.

## Non-Covered Services

Sometimes an insurance company will deny authorization or payment for a certain test or treatment because your insurance plan outright does not cover that particular test or treatment. These types of denials are challenging to appeal because the insurance company is not claiming that the medical care is unnecessary or experimental. They are simply stating that the insurance policy that you signed up for does not include coverage of this particular test or treatment. Essentially, even if the insurance company agrees that the proposed medical care is necessary and appropriate, they still deny coverage because this particular item is not on their menu of covered services. It is still possible (but challenging) to appeal for coverage, asking that the insurance company make an exception in your case.

## Open Enrollment, Changing Insurance Companies

Most employers provide a narrow window of time (a few weeks or months) during which you can change your health insurance coverage. Be aware of these deadlines, which are usually near the end of the calendar year. You may also be able to change your insurance at other times, such as upon getting married or having a child. Do your homework to figure out which insurance plan is best for you and your family.

For example, if you need tailbone injections or pelvic floor physical therapy, then find out which of the available insurance plans provide the best coverage for these. If your most pressing medical condition involves treatment by one particular physician specialist or one particular physical therapy center, then investigate which insurance plans cover the specific clinicians that you desire. Or choose a plan that allows for adequate coverage of out-of-network clinicians.

Be sure to compare not only the costs of your monthly premiums, but also your own out-of-pocket costs (such as your annual out-of-network deductible and copays).

## Out-of-Pocket Expenses

Different insurance plans will result in differences in your own out-of-pocket expenses. Some plans will have a yearly out-of-pocket deductible amount. For example, early in the calendar year you may be paying 100 percent of the costs for seeing an out-of-network physician. But part way through the calendar year you may have made enough out-of-pocket payments that your insurance company starts helping to pay for subsequent expenses. For example, if you had a $1,000 out-of-pocket deductible, then you will pay the first $1,000 of certain medical expenses. After that, your insurance company may pay 80 percent of the additional costs. Look at the details, since each plan varies.

In general, this means that by later in the calendar year, many people have already paid their out-of-pocket deductible for the year. If further medical services are needed, then it is to the patient's advantage to obtain those services while the insurance company is now responsible for a large portion of the payments. Do this before the end of the current calendar year, because on January 1 you will go back to paying 100 percent of the expenses toward your next year's out-of-pocket deductible.

Save your receipts and talk with a tax accountant, since medical expenses may be deductible from your state and/or federal taxes. Talk with your employer's payroll office about setting up a "medical flexible spending account." This allows you to avoid paying income tax on money that you set aside to pay your medical bills during the upcoming calendar year.

## International Patients

People from other countries who travel to the United States for medical care typically pay for their medical care here at the time of service. You may be able to submit your receipts for reimbursement from the health insurance plan in your home country. Details vary by country.

## Car Insurance and Workers' Compensation Insurance

If you injured your tailbone during an car accident, then your medical care should be covered under your automobile insurance.

This part of your car insurance is sometimes called "Personal Injury Protection" (PIP). Be sure to keep any letters from your car insurance company and know your insurance claim number.

If you injured your tailbone at work, then your medical care should be covered by workers' compensation insurance. If your workers' compensation insurance company does not have a specialist with expertise in evaluating and treating tailbone pain, you can request the insurance company to authorize your getting treated someplace that does have that expertise.

Automobile injuries and on-the-job injuries often involve lawsuits, which will be discussed in Chapter 30: *Legal Cases for Tailbone Injuries.*

## Free Bonus for You

For your free printable form to help you track your interactions with your insurance company, go to: **TailboneDoctor.com/forms**

# Legal Cases for Tailbone Injuries

## Barbara's Story

When Barbara slipped on a wet floor while shopping at her local grocery store, she severely injured her tailbone. It was still painful one year later. Her injury resulted in multiple medical bills and extensive lost time from work. She consulted an attorney to begin a lawsuit against the grocery store. But, unfortunately, she and her lawyer found that her medical records failed to provide adequate evidence of the tailbone injury. The imaging reports and physical exam notes had failed to explicitly address the tailbone findings.

Barbara came for evaluation at our Tailbone Pain Center, where review of those actual images revealed that they had not even included the tailbone. New x-rays and an MRI were ordered, focusing on the optimal images for tailbone evaluation. Results provided clear and objective evidence that her coccyx had been fractured at exactly the site where she was reporting persistent pain. This evidence greatly strengthened her legal case, leading to her successfully winning her lawsuit.

Some people with tailbone injuries need to navigate not only the medical system but also the legal system. For example, if your tailbone injury happened at work, or during an auto accident, or due to negligence of another person or business, you may need to take legal steps to obtain financial compensation for your medical care and lost work time, as well as for your pain and suffering.

## Legal Challenges: Imaging Studies

One difficulty with legal cases involving tailbone injuries is that you need to have appropriate medical testing done to document the injury. Most tailbone injuries will fail to be adequately detected by standard sacrum/coccyx x-rays, lumbar MRIs, lumbosacral MRIs, or pelvic MRIs.

**People with tailbone injuries face multiple challenges within the legal system.**

These various diagnostic tests require specific modifications to optimize their ability to detect coccyx injuries. These modifications include coned-down x-rays, sitting x-rays, and thin midline sagittal views of the coccyx on MRI or CT scans.

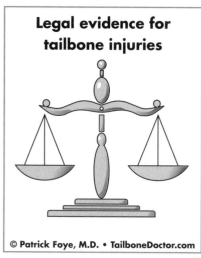

**Legal evidence for tailbone injuries**

© Patrick Foye, M.D. • TailboneDoctor.com

If the imaging studies are not done properly, the results will fail to detect your coccyx injury. Unfortunately, that will weaken your legal case, since the available evidence would suggest that perhaps there was no tailbone injury at all. Having the proper testing done is crucial. (See Chapter 16: *Medical Tests for Tailbone Pain*.)

## Legal Challenges: Clinical Expertise

If your treating physicians do not have experience, training, skills, and expertise in treating tailbone injuries, then they may not order the diagnostic studies properly. Those doctors also may fail to personally review the images or may fail to perform a careful or thorough physical examination of the tailbone region. Further, the physicians may fail to adequately document all of the imaging results, physical exam findings, and the interpretation as to how these findings do (or do not) match with your history of tailbone trauma.

## Legal Challenges: Treatment

Many doctors, lawyers, judges, and insurance companies may be unaware of the currently available treatments for coccyx injuries.

This can be problematic for you if any or all of those parties are seeking to close (that is, shutdown) your medical and legal case before all appropriate treatments have been considered and provided. Once your legal case is settled or closed, you may have difficulty getting coverage later for treatments that should have been tried sooner.

## Summary

People with tailbone injuries face multiple challenges within the legal system. These challenges include obtaining evidence clearly showing the tailbone injury, establishing that the injury was actually caused by the specific traumatic incident in question, and obtaining compensation to cover you for the related medical tests, treatments, medications, and for your pain and suffering. Overcoming these challenges may require working closely with your lawyer and with a physician experienced in successfully handling these challenges specifically related to tailbone injuries.

## Free Bonus for You

For your free printable checklist to help you document your tailbone pain in a legal case, go to: **TailboneDoctor.com/forms**

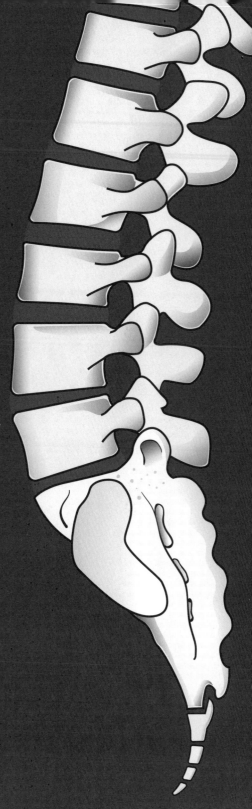

PART FOUR

# Book
# Summary

# CHAPTER 31

# Take Home Points

Congratulations on having read *Tailbone Pain Relief Now!*

These *Take Home Points* serve only as a very brief summary. You have truly covered a LOT of material on tailbone pain. From the information in this book, you have learned more about tailbone pain than probably 99.9 percent of physicians! If I could give you a diploma from a mini-med school for the coccyx, I would gladly bestow it upon you.

You've learned about the symptoms of tailbone pain, especially how tailbone pain worsens with sitting and sometimes during the initial moments of going from sitting to standing.

You've learned about the psychological stigma sometimes attached to tailbone pain, and how to overcome that stigma by empowering yourself with knowledge, action, and open communication.

You've discovered the variety of common causes of tailbone pain, including unstable joints of the tailbone (dynamic instability, which is excessive joint movement while sitting), fractures, dislocations, bone spurs, arthritis, abnormal coccyx positions, sympathetic nervous system pain, cancer, infections, and more.

You've learned about the most helpful diagnostic tests for tailbone pain, including x-rays done while sitting, as well as MRI studies, CT scans, and other tests. You've learned that these studies are only helpful if they are done properly, so that they very explicitly focus on the tailbone.

Beyond testing, you've learned about the scope of available treatment options with tailbone pain, including cushions, medications, manipulation, various injections, and surgery.

More important than just the information that you have learned, hopefully you've had a chance to actively apply this fund of knowledge so that you can obtain the best possible medical care for your tailbone pain. Knowledge *without action* will *not* make the positive difference that you are seeking. This book is meant to empower you as you actively seek the tests and treatments necessary to provide you with the relief that you desire and deserve.

The road to recovery often has speed bumps, potholes, detours, and obstacles. Hopefully *Tailbone Pain Relief Now!* has given you a useful roadmap showing you how to navigate through the tests and treatments that you need. My heart goes out to you as you travel on this journey.

Medical care is continually advancing. To discover the latest information and blog postings on tailbone pain, or to arrange to meet me in person, join me online at **TailboneDoctor.com.**

## Free Bonus for You

For your free printable copies of all of the various checklists, forms and step-by-step guides related to tailbone pain, go to:

**TailboneDoctor.com/forms**

# Come for Medical Care from Dr. Foye

At his Tailbone Pain Center, Dr. Foye treats patients who come from around the country and around the world.

To come for an in-person evaluation by Dr. Foye, start by visiting his website at **TailboneDoctor.com** or call: 973-972-2802. Or simply send an email to: **Tailbone.Pain@gmail.com** (an automatic reply will instantly email you a link containing information on how to come see Dr. Foye).

You can also follow Dr. Foye and the Tailbone Pain Center online at the following sites:

 https://facebook.com/pages/Tailbone-Pain-Center-Coccyx-Pain-Center/82665772981

 https://youtube.com/user/TailbonePainDoctor

 LinkedIn http://linkedin.com/pub/patrick-foye-md/a5/9bb/117

 http://pinterest.com/doctorfoye/

 https://twitter.com/TailboneDoctor

# Testimonials from Dr. Foye's Patients

**Dear Dr. Foye ...** Thanks to you I can sit again without pain. My only regret is that I didn't come to see you sooner.

—**Betty G.**, administrative assistant, Massachusetts

**Dear Dr. Foye ...** I finally feel that I am in the correct place with the correct doctor! I am so glad I found you.

—**Helen B.**, retail sales person, Maryland

**Dear Dr. Foye ...** Words cannot express my gratitude for your excellent care and attention. I am like a new person!

—**Daniel A.**, airline pilot, California

**Dear Dr. Foye ...** You fixed my tailbone years ago and I wanted to let you know it's still holding and made a vast difference in my quality of life. Thank you!     —**Sandra J.**, research scientist, Texas

**Dear Dr. Foye ...** I truly appreciate you taking the time to answer all of my questions and share your knowledge. I feel that I will have more of a normal life thanks to you! God bless you!

—**Carol M.**, food-service worker, New Jersey

**Dear Dr. Foye ...** Thanks so much for all of your help during this most difficult time of my life! I am almost 100% better now, looking for a job and back in school. All the best to you!

—**Andrew R.**, graduate student, Arizona

**Dear Dr. Foye ...** What can I say but thank you for the care you gave me. You and your medical team are so special to me. I can sit anywhere now and that makes me so happy!

—**Sharon S.**, mother and personal trainer, Pennsylvania

**Dear Dr. Foye ...** I am writing to offer my sincere thanks to you and your team for your extraordinary care you gave me. From the friendliness and efficiency of the front desk staff, to your on-site x-ray services and information—all aspects of my visit were terrific. It is a rare experience to visit with a doctor who is so caring and committed to his patients.          —**Ruth P.**, secretary, New York

# About the Author

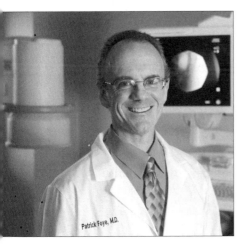

Patrick Foye, M.D.

**Dr. Patrick Foye** is a native of New Jersey, where he earned a bachelor's degree in biology and chemistry from Drew University. He then attended New Jersey Medical School, where he received his M.D. in 1992.

Dr. Foye did his internship in internal medicine at St. Barnabas Medical Center in Livingston, New Jersey, where he was named "Intern of the Year" and "Most Compassionate Resident."

He did his residency training in Physical Medicine and Rehabilitation (PM&R) at Northwestern University's prestigious Rehabilitation Institute of Chicago, where he was Chief Resident.

Dr. Foye became a faculty member at New Jersey Medical School in 1996, where he founded the Tailbone Pain Center. He has obtained multiple board certifications, including in PM&R and pain management.

As a medical school professor, Dr. Foye has written extensively on the topics of pain, musculoskeletal medicine, and tailbone injuries. He has published more than 200 medical research articles, book chapters, review articles, conference abstracts, and other medical publications. At Rutgers New Jersey Medical School, Dr. Foye has been inducted into the Masters Educators Guild, and has received the university's Excellence in Teaching Award. He has taught over 800 lectures and workshops for medical students, resident physicians, medical doctors, physical therapists, and other healthcare providers. The American Academy of Physical Medicine and Rehabilitation (AAPM&R) has honored him with the national Distinguished Clinician Award. Dr. Foye has also been named as one of "America's Top Physicians."

Dr. Foye and his research have been covered extensively in the media, including: *Time* magazine, *National Public Radio* (NPR), Fox News, the *British Broadcasting Corporation* (BBC), *Regis and Kathy Lee,* and many others. *USA Today* named Dr. Foye as one of the nation's "Most Influential Doctors."

With many years of experience and expertise as Founder and Medical Director of the Tailbone Pain Center, Dr. Foye has provided thousands of evaluations and treatments for patients with tailbone pain.

For more information, or to schedule an evaluation, go to Dr. Foye's website: **TailboneDoctor.com**

# Acknowledgments

**I am immensely grateful** to the countless people who have contributed to my medical and personal knowledge and skills during more than 25 years of medical training and practice.

First and foremost, I thank my patients. They have been my greatest teachers. Although I have read hundreds of medical articles and book chapters about tailbone pain, my thousands of patients have taught me far more. I am honored by the trust you place in me, and it is immensely gratifying to be able to help so many of you. You inspire me to be the best physician possible and to educate others regarding tailbone pain.

I also thank my patients for advising and motivating me to make coccyx information available by creating:

- my website **TailboneDoctor.com** (Mr. H.H.),

- YouTube videos (channel: **youtube.com/user/ TailbonePainDoctor**),

- a Facebook page (**facebook.com/pages/Tailbone-Pain-Center-Coccyx-Pain-Center/82665772981**),

- Twitter (**@TailboneDoctor**),

- Pinterest (**pinterest.com/doctorfoye**), and

- this book, *Tailbone Pain Relief Now!*

I thank my wife Sarah, son Adam, parents Mary & Martin Foye, and siblings (Maureen, Marty, Mike, and Sean) for their love and support.

I thank my physician role models, including Drs. Todd P. Stitik, Boqing Chen, John R. Bach, Elliot J. Roth, James A. Sliwa, Dennis P. Quinlan, Susan G. Mautone, and Thomas J. Stack.

I thank my office staff Grace Sia, Marisol Salva, Carol Dunne, Brian DaSilva, Doreen Muhammad, and Geoff Seeger, for their years of hard work and dedication in helping me and the patients seen at my medical practice.

I thank the medical researchers whose publications have helped me immensely, especially Dr. Jean-Yves Maigne for his wonderful medical research on coccyx pain.

I thank Jon Miles, a retired physicist in England, who has created valuable resources for people suffering from tailbone pain and the doctors who treat them.

I thank the thousands of medical students, physical therapy students, resident physicians, fellows, medical office volunteers, and colleagues who I have taught over the years. Teaching something is the best way to learn it well. Also, your questions prompt me to explore new alternatives and deeper levels of understanding.

I thank the centronuclear/titin myopathy team, including Alan Beggs, Paul and Alison Frase, Pam and Gary Scoggin, Sarah Jajesnica Foye, and so many others, for showing how to make a positive difference for a rare condition.

I'm grateful to Landmark Education's Jessica Licata, Jerry Roberts, Jack Licata, Rock & Rita Fiore, and others, for years of motivation, transformation, and breakthroughs. I thank inspirational podcasters Sam Crowley (*Every Day is Saturday*) and Matt Theriault (*the Do-Over Guy*). Thanks to consultant David Santoriello.

I also thank the Center for Plain Language and my book publishing team, including Judith Briles (The Book Shepherd), my editors, illustrator, design team, printer, and book distributor.

# Bibliography/References

**Over the past two decades,** I have read many hundreds of medical journal articles on tailbone pain. While it would not be practical to list every such article here, this bibliography contains many of my most important sources in writing this book. This bibliography also includes many of my own previous publications on the topic of tailbone pain—works from which I have drawn and expanded upon to create this book.

Alo GO, Eisenstein SM, Darby A. The sacro-coccygeal joint in coccydynia. *The Journal of Bone and Joint Surgery.* British volume. 1998;80-B(2S):196.

Atim A, Ergin A, Bilgiç S, Deniz S, Kurt E. Pulsed radiofrequency in the treatment of coccygodynia. *Agri.* 2011 Jan;23(1):1-6.

Balain B, Eisenstein SM, Alo GO, et al. Coccygectomy for coccydynia: case series and review of literature. *Spine.* 2006 Jun;31(13):E414-20.

Borgia CA. Coccydynia: its diagnosis and treatment. *Military medicine.* 1964 Apr;129:335-8.

Buttaci CJ, Foye PM, Stitik TP. Coccydynia Successfully Treated with Ganglion Impar Blocks: A Case Series. *American Journal of Physical Medicine and Rehabilitation.* 2005;84(3):218.

Doursounian L, Maigne JY, Faure F, Chatellier G. *International orthopaedics.* 2004 Jun;28(3):176-9.

Eisenstein SM, Darby AJ, Cassar-Pullicino, et al. Sacrococcygeal Pain and Pathology: Coccydynia Revisited. *The Journal of bone and joint surgery.* British. 2000; 82-B(Supplement-II):98-99.

Fortin JD, Falco FJ. The Fortin Finger Test: an Indicator of Sacroiliac Pain. *The American Journal of Orthopedics.* 1997 Jul;26(7):477-80.

Foye PM, Brubaker M, Kamanga-Sollo G, et al.. Banana boat Tailbone Trauma: 100% Complete Listhesis, a Dynamic Dislocation. *American Journal of Physical Medicine & Rehabilitation.* 2011 April; 90(4):a25.

Foye PM, Brubaker M, Kamanga-Sollo G. Sit-To-Stand Exacerbation of Coccyx Pain As a Predictor of Coccygeal Dynamic Instability Versus Bone Spurs. *American Journal of Physical Medicine & Rehabilitation.* 2011 April; 90(4):

Foye PM, Buttaci CJ, Stitik TP, et al. Successful injection for coccyx pain. *American Journal of Physical Medicine & Rehabilitation.* 2006 Sep;85(9):783-4.

Foye PM, Buttaci CJ. Coccyx Pain. In: Plantz SH, eMedicine: Physical Medicine and Rehabilitation. San Francisco: eMedicine; 2007. *emedicine.com/pmr/topic242.htm*

Foye PM, Desai RD. MRI, CT scan, and dynamic radiographs for coccydynia. *Joint, Bone, Spine: Revue du Rhumatisme.* 2014 May;81(3):280.

Foye PM, Enriquez R, Kamrava E. Seated MRI for Patients with Tailbone Pain: a Case Series. *PM R,* 2009 Sept;1(9):S223-S224.

Foye PM, *et al.* Psychological versus Physical Pain Descriptors in Patients with Tailbone Pain. *American Journal of Physical Medicine & Rehabilitation.* 2010 April;89(4):S32-3.

Foye PM, Kamrava E, Enriquez R. Tailbone Pain Associated with a Keel-Shaped Coccyx: a Case Series. *PM R,* 2009 Sept;1(9):S176-S177.

Foye PM, Kamrava E, Enriquez R. Tailbone Pain from Coccyx Injuries on Water Slides: a Case Series. *PM R,* 2009 Sept;1(9):S177.

Foye PM, Kumar S. CT Morphology and Morphometry of the normal adult coccyx. *European Spine Journal.* 2013 Nov 30.

Foye PM, Patel SL. Paracoccygeal Corkscrew Approach to Ganglion Impar Injections for Tailbone Pain. *Pain Practice* (the official journal of the World Institute of Pain). 2009 July-Aug;9(4):317-321

Foye PM, Sanderson SO, Smith JA. Coccyx Cushions for Tailbone Pain: Donut Cushions Versus Wedge Cushions. *American Journal of Physical Medicine and Rehabilitation.* 2009 Mar;88(3):S56.

Foye PM, Schoenherr L, Kim JH. Coccydynia (Coccyx Pain) after Colonoscopy. *American Journal of Physical Medicine and Rehabilitation.* 2008 Mar;87(3):S36.

Foye PM, Shupper P, Wendel I. Coccyx fractures treated with intranasal calcitonin. *Pain Physician.* 2014 Mar-Apr;17(2):E229-33.

Foye PM, Smith JA, Sanderson SO. Cookie-Bite Coccyx: Retained Coccygeal Fragment after Coccygectomy. *American Journal of Physical Medicine and Rehabilitation.* 2009 Mar;88(3):S56.

Foye PM, Stitik TP. Diagnostic Ultrasound in a Patient with Tailbone Pain: Detecting Coccygeal Dislocation/Listhesis but Failing to Detect an Avulsion Fracture of the Coccyx. *American Journal of Physical Medicine & Rehabilitation.* 2010 April;89(4):S33.

Foye PM, Vora MN. Sacrococcygeal cornua as zygapophysial joints. *Anatomical Science International.* 2014 Sep;89(4):266.

Foye PM. A New Diagnostic Test for Coccyx Pain (Tailbone Pain): Seated MRI. *American Journal of Physical Medicine and Rehabilitation.* 2008 Mar;87(3):S36.

Foye PM. Anal Nerve Risks with Paracoccygeal Lumbosacral Fixation. *Surgical and Radiologic Anatomy: SRA.* Oct. 2010. 32(8):805.

Foye PM. Causality of concomitant coccyx pain and lumbar pain. The Journal of Bone and Joint Surgery. British volume. 2010 Dec. Published online: *http://bjj.boneandjoint.org.uk/content/ 92-B/12/1622/reply#jbjsbr_el_5412*

Foye PM. Coccydynia (Coccyx Pain) Caused by Chordoma. *Int Orthop.* 2007 Jun;31(3):427.

Foye PM. Coccyx Pain and MRI: Precoccygeal epidermal inclusion cyst. *Singapore medical journal.* 2010 May;51(5):450.

Foye PM. Coccyx Pain Diagnostic Workup: Necessity of MRI in Detecting Malignancy Presenting with Tailbone Pain. *American Journal of Physical Medicine & Rehabilitation.* 2010 April;89(4):S33.

Foye PM. Dextrose prolotherapy for recalcitrant coccygodynia fractures. *Journal of Orthopaedic Surgery* (Hong Kong). 2008 Aug;16(2):270.

Foye PM. Finding the cause of coccydynia (coccyx pain). *The Journal of Bone and Joint Surgery.* British volume. 2007 Jan; online: *http://jbjs.org.uk/cgi/eletters/88-B/10/1388.*

Foye PM. Ganglion Impar Blocks for Chronic Pelvic and Coccyx Pain. *Pain Physician.* 2007 Nov;10(6):780-1.

Foye PM. Ganglion Impar Blocks via Coccygeal versus Sacrococcygeal Joints. *Regional Anesthesia and Pain Medicine.* 2008 May-Jun; 33(3):279-80.

Foye PM. Ganglion impar injection techniques for coccydynia (coccyx pain) and pelvic pain. *Anesthesiology.* 2007 May; 106(5):1062-3.

Foye PM. Ganglion Impar Pulsed Radiofrequency for Coccyx Pain. *Journal of Pain and Symptom Management.* April 2011. 41(4):e11-12.

Foye PM. Imaging Studies Detecting Retrorectal Tumors. *Turkish Journal of Gastroenterology.* 2009 Jan;20(1):81.

Foye PM. New approaches to Ganglion Impar Blocks, via Coccygeal Joints. *Regional Anesthesia and Pain Medicine.* 2007 May-Jun;32(3):269.

Foye PM. Reasons to Delay or Avoid Coccygectomy for Coccyx Pain. *Injury.* 2007 Nov;38(11):1328-1329.

Foye PM. Safe ganglion Impar blocks for visceral and coccyx pain. *Techniques in Regional Anesthesia and Pain Management.* 2008 Apr;12(2):122-123.

Foye PM. Stigma Against Patients with Coccyx Pain. *Pain medicine.* 2010 Dec;11(12):1872.

Foye PM. Tailbone Pain (Coccydynia) Treated with Phenol Chemical Ablation of Somatic Nerves at the Posterior Coccyx. *American Journal of Physical Medicine and Rehabilitation.* 2009 Mar;88(3):S56-57.

Gopal H, McCrory C. Coccygodynia treated by pulsed radio frequency treatment to the Ganglion of Impar: a case series. *Journal of Back and Musculoskeletal Rehabilitation.* 2014 Feb;27(3):349-54

Hodges SD, Eck JC, Humphreys SC. A treatment and outcomes analysis of patients with coccydynia. *The Spine Journal:* official journal of the North American Spine Society. 2004 Mar-Apr; 4(2):138-40.

Howorth B. The painful coccyx. *Clinical orthopaedics.* 1959; 14:145-60.

Hughes SV, Pietroni D. Stigma and the perception of bodily parts: Implications for help seeking. *Pelviperineology.* 2014 March;33(1):29-31.

Kabbara AI. Transsacrococcygeal ganglion impar block for postherpetic neuralgia. *Anesthesiology.* 2005 Jul;103(1):211-2.

Kerr EE, Benson D, Schrot RJ. Coccygectomy for chronic refractory coccygodynia: clinical case series and literature review. *Journal of neurosurgery, Spine.* 2011 May;14(5):654-63.

Kuthuru M, Kabbara AI, Oldenburg P, et al. Coccygeal pain relief after transsacrococcygeal block of the ganglion Impar under fluoroscopy: a case report. *Archives of Physical Medicine and Rehabilitation.* 2003 Sep;84(9):E24.

Lercher K, Foye PM. Heterotopic Ossification of the Coccyx as a Post-Operative Complication of Coccygectomy. *American Journal of Physical Medicine & Rehabilitation.* 2011 April; 90(4): 87-88.

Liang CW, Foye PM, Sorenson MK. Low Incidence of Vascular Uptake in Ganglion Impar Injections for Coccydynia (Coccyx Pain). *American Journal of Physical Medicine and Rehabilitation.* 2007 Apr;86(4):S104.

Maigne JY, Chatellier G, Faou ML, et al. The treatment of chronic coccydynia with intrarectal manipulation: a randomized controlled study. *Spine.* 2006 Aug;31(18):E621-7.

Maigne JY, Doursounian L, Chatellier G. Causes and mechanisms of common coccydynia: role of body mass index and coccygeal trauma. *Spine.* 2000 Dec;25(23):3072-9.

Maigne JY, Guedj S, Fautrel B. Coccygodynia: value of dynamic lateral x-ray films in sitting position. *Rev Rhum Mal Osteoartic.* 1992 Nov;59(11):728-31.

Maigne JY, Tamalet B. Standardized radiologic protocol for the study of common coccygodynia and characteristics of the lesions observed in the sitting position. Clinical elements differentiating luxation, hypermobility, and normal mobility. *Spine.* 1996 Nov; 21(22):2588-93.

Maigne, JY, Chatellier G. Comparison of three manual coccydynia treatments: a pilot study. *Spine.* 2001;26(20):E479-483.

Maigne, JY, Guedj S, et al.. Idiopathic coccygodynia. Lateral roentgenograms in the sitting position and coccygeal discography. *Spine.* 1994;19(8):930-934.

Maigne, JY, Lagauche D, et al. Instability of the coccyx in coccydynia. *The Journal of Bone and Joint Surgery.* British volume. 2000;82(7):1038-1041.

Nathan ST, Fisher BE, Roberts CS. Coccydynia: a review of pathoanatomy, aetiology, treatment and outcome. *The Journal of Bone and Joint Surgery.* British volume. 2010 Dec;92(12):1622-7.

Oh CS, Chung IH, Ji HJ, *et al.* Clinical implications of topographic anatomy on the ganglion impar. *Anesthesiology.* 2004 Jul; 101(1):249-50.

Pennekamp PH, Kraft CN, Stütz A, et al. Coccygectomy for coccygodynia: does pathogenesis matter? *The Journal of Trauma.* 2005 Dec;59(6):1414-9.

Plancarte R, Amescua C, Patt RB, *et al.* Presacral blockade of the ganglion of Walther (ganglion Impar). *Anesthesiology.* 1990;73(3a):A751.

Reig E, Abejón D, Del Pozo C, *et al.* Thermocoagulation of the ganglion impar or ganglion of walther: description of a modified approach. Preliminary results in chronic, nononcological pain. *Pain Practice:* the official journal of World Institute of Pain. 2005 Jun;5(2):103-10.

Rhee M, Foye PM, Tung D. Coccydynia (Coccyx Pain) due to Dynamic Instability of the Tailbone: A Case Report. *Archives of Physical Medicine and Rehabilitation.* 2007 Sep;88(9): E36.

Richette P, Maigne JY, Bardin T. Coccydynia related to calcium crystal deposition. *Spine.* 2008 Aug;33(17):E620-3.

Stein A., *Heal Pelvic Pain: A Proven Stretching, Strengthening, and Nutrition Program for Relieving Pain, Incontinence, IBS, and Other Symptoms without Surgery.* New York: McGraw-Hill, 2009. Print.

Wood KB, Mehbod AA. Operative treatment for coccygodynia. *Journal of Spinal Disorders & Techniques.* 2004 Dec;17(6):511-5.

Wray CC, Easom S, Hoskinson J. Coccydynia. Aetiology and treatment. *The Journal of Bone and Joint Surgery.* British volume. 1991 Mar;73(2):335-8.

# Index

## A

ablation. *See* nerve ablation
antibiotics 96–97, 99–102, 111
anus 19, 23, 36, 91, 102, 108, 111, 113, 130, 134–36, 167, 169–70, 173, 196, 199, 207
anxiety 23, 25, 26, 28, 163
arthritis 31, 37–38, 41, 60, 71–73, 78-9, 109, 130, 146, 153, 163, 183, 187, 189

## B

baby 53-4, 77, 135, 154, 215-16, 217–18, 220–22
back pain, low 103-114, 124, 180, 208-9
bacteria 95-6, 99–101, 197
bedsores 93–94, 100
birth canal 53–54, 77–78, 217–18, 220
bloodstream 95, 98–100, 128
bloodwork 97, 99, 116, 130
bones 16, 30, 32, 40–42, 44–47, 52, 56–57, 59–63, 65–67, 71–73, 89–90, 94–97, 99–102, 117–18, 127–29
chip of 52
coccygeal 19, 30, 33–35, 36, 41–43, 44–47, 52–56, 62–64, 68, 73, 94-5, 117, 119–20, 124, 127, 147, 169,172, 183–84, 187-8, 190, 192, 210, 216–17, 224
dislocated. *See* dislocations
fractured. *See* fractures
ischial 16, 114, 177
lumbar vertebral 106–7
pelvic 36, 217
pubic 116–17, 134
spinal 30, 101
vertebral 30, 101, 106–7
bone scans 89–90, 97–98, 127–29, 200
bone spur 37–38, 65–70, 117, 134, 145, 172, 184, 187, 216, 218, 220
bowel movements 20, 53, 75-6, 77-78, 87–88, 113, 130, 135, 164, 167
breastfeeding 154, 221–22
bricks 41, 42, 45–46, 60–61, 156
buttock pain 18, 21, 29, 103, 105–7, 109–11, 113, 180
buttocks 16, 23, 53, 58, 103–4, 110, 114, 147, 156–57, 166–67, 177, 180

## C

cancer 38, 85–92, 101–2, 115, 123–24, 126–28, 130-31, 135–37, 142, 164, 196, 200, 213
bone 85–86, 128
rectal 87–89, 130, 135
underlying 88–89, 91, 187
CD, of x-ray images 211, 211
CD, of MRI images 126
cervix 87–89, 123, 135
chair 27, 39, 68, 73, 76, 78, 114, 121, 147, 155–58, 167
childbirth 77–78, 135, 215–18, 220-2
children 23, 132, 202, 223–26
chordoma, 85–87
coccydynia. *See* tailbone pain
coccygeal. *See* tailbone
coccygeal dynamic instability 39, 40, 42–44, 46, 48-9, 115, 171, 188, 224
coccygectomy. *See* surgery to remove the tailbone
coccygeus muscles 19, 35, 134
coccygodynia. *See* tailbone pain
coccyx. *See* tailbone

bone, number   34
fracture. *See* fractures
joints. *See* joints
movement   119–20
pain. *See* tailbone pain
x-rays. *See* x-rays
colon   75, 85, 91, 123, 130, 132,
   135–36, 211, 213
colon cancer   131, 135
colonoscopy   75, 91, 130–31, 135–36
Complex Regional Pain Syndrome.
   *See* CRPS
computer CD of images   126, 203,
   211
constipation   77, 164–65, 181, 222
consultations, 20, 92, 102, 124, 131,
   132-33, 135, 137, 212
CPT code   232
CRPS (Complex Regional Pain Syndrome)   81, 83
CT scans   54-5, 63, 68, 72, 89–90, 94,
   98, 115-16, 122–24, 183, 187, 199,
   208, 210, 219, 225, 240
cushions   49, 70, 74, 121, 137,
   151–58, 187, 221, 226
   doughnut   151–52
   ring   152–53
   wedge   151–54


**D**
delivery. *See* childbirth
depression   25–26, 28, 163, 165
diagnostic coccyx injections   186
dislocations   37–38, 45, 58–64, 124,
   183–84, 190, 218
dynamic instability   18–19, 24, 37–
   39, 40–44, 46–48, 58, 115, 120, 171,
   188, 190, 224

**E**
excessive tailbone movement   18,
   46–47, 120, 184, 190, 224
exercises,   26, 175–76, 178–80
extension   42–44, 46, 66, 95, 109,
   172


**F**
fluoroscopy   33, 164, 181–83, 185,
   187
fractures of the tailbone   25, 32, 37,
   38, 40, 51–58, 60-62, 64, 78, 124,
   164-66, 172, 183, 218


**G**
ganglia   36, 79, 82
ganglion Impar   36, 83, 185–87
   hyperactivity   83
genital region   20, 24, 112–13, 116,
   134, 136, 177


**I**
imaging studies   33–34, 54–55, 63,
   68, 69, 72, 78, 85, 89, 91, 97, 115–30,
   187, 199, 200, 203-4, 208, 210,
   212–13, 240
immobilization   56–57, 63
infection   93–102, 124, 127, 130, 136,
   187, 192, 195–98, 200, 221
   bone   93–97, 99–101, 124,
   127–28, 200
   sacrococcygeal   95
   symptoms   95
   TB (tuberculosis)   101, 130
inflammation   71, 73, 97–98, 107–8,
   115, 124, 136, 156, 160–63, 166,
   182–84, 186

injections   74, 79, 82–83, 108, 133,
    137, 141-43, 49, 145, 158, 162-63,
    181–93, 195, 198, 200, 204, 219,
    230, 231, 235
  benefits   190–91
  blind   182–83
  diagnostic   186
  image guidance   181–83, 185, 187
  steroid   187
  test   109, 186–88
instability   18-19, 24, 37-9, 40–42, 46,
    78, 115, 120, 153, 171
insurance, medical   227-37
  appeals   229, 233–35
  company   204, 213, 227–37, 241
  coverage   231, 234–35, 241
  denials   227, 231–34
  out-of-network   228–29
  plans,   228–30, 234–35
  pre-authorizations   231–33
intestines   81, 161, 163–64, 191
ischial bones,   16, 33, 113–14, 177
ischial bursitis   106, 113–14, 156


J
joints   18, 30-1, 34, 40–41, 43-4, 53,
    59–60, 62, 72-73, 77, 104, 109, 120,
    166, 184, 188–89, 216–17, 224
  tailbone   34, 72–73, 171, 183, 190,
    217, 224
  unstable   18–19, 24, 37, 40, 49,
    171–72, 188, 224
joint spaces   42, 46–47, 60, 72–73,
    117, 183–84, 188, 190


L
leaning   18, 68, 103-4, 109, 114,
    118-19, 145–47, 178, 216
legal cases   239–41
leg pain   82, 103–4, 106, 108–10, 114,
    156

ligaments   33, 35–36, 42, 61, 63,
    112, 132–33, 170, 188–89, 196,
    198, 217
  anterior sacrococcygeal   35, 61
  in tailbone dislocations   61
listhesis   44–47, 120
local anesthetics   79, 82–83, 109,
    185–88
lumbar radiculopathy   108–10
lumbar spine   30, 106–9, 115, 118,
    125


M
malignancy. See cancer
manipulation   140, 169–73
medical specialists   101, 132–33, 135,
    137, 212
medications   23, 26, 49, 70, 74, 133,
    137, 141–42, 145, 159–65, 167, 175,
    181–82, 184–87, 191–93, 195, 198,
    200, 215, 222, 231
  nonsteroidal. See NSAIDs
  opioid. See opioids
  over-the-counter   191
  pain   27, 142, 159, 164, 191, 215,
    222, 231, 241
MRI   32–33, 54-5, 63, 68, 72, 75, 89–
    90, 98–99, 107, 123–27, 187, 199,
    207–10, 230, 225, 232, 239–40
muscles   19, 33, 35–36, 58, 61, 66, 79,
    81, 102, 112-13, 132–34, 142, 166,
    170-1, 176, 180, 184, 188, 196, 198-
    99, 217


N
nerve ablation   133, 186–88, 192,
    198
nerve blocks   79, 82-3, 133, 185, 189,
    198
nerve destruction. See nerve ablation

nerve pain   79, 106, 110, 165, 186
  relief, 133
nerves   24, 36, 67, 79–80, 82, 108,
  112, 185–87, 192
  sciatic   110, 156
NSAIDs   133, 160–63, 166, 219


**O**

opioids   164–65, 222
osteoarthritis   71–73, 189
osteomyelitis   93, 95, 97–98, 124,
  127–28, 197–98


**P**

pain
  after coccygectomy   95, 198-99
  chronic   26–28, 81, 112, 164
  fracture   165
  joint   103, 106, 109
  lumbosacral   208–9
  musculoskeletal   18, 79, 104, 113,
    160, 183, 186
  pelvic   24-5, 27, 123, 135, 225
  relieve   133, 166, 222, 231
  sympathetically-maintained
    36, 81-3, 185
painkillers. See medications
pain medications. See medications
pelvic
  contents   112–13
  floor   33, 35, 112–13, 133–35,
    169–70, 173, 180, 196, 198–99,
    200, 235
  floor pain   112–13, 135, 180
  floor prolapse   198–200
  MRI   89, 125–26, 232, 240
  organs   35, 90, 123–24, 133,
    198–99, 213, 232
  pain syndrome   24, 27, 113, 135
  region   24, 89–90, 104, 108, 124,
    167, 219

persistent pain   81, 196, 198–200,
  239
physical therapist (PT)   110, 113,
  133–34, 142, 173, 180, 204
physicians
  out-of-network   228-29, 233, 235
  pain management   113, 132–33
pilonidal cysts   111
piriformis muscle   18, 103-4,
  106, 110
  pain   103, 110
Platelet-rich plasma (PRP)   188-89
pre-authorization. See insurance
pregnancy   53, 78, 135, 202, 215–17,
  219, 221–22
pregnant women   77, 216, 219
pressure
  direct   121, 131, 148–49, 153, 176,
    178–79, 226
  excessive   156
pressure ulcers. See bedsores
prolapse   113, 198–99, 200
prostate cancer   87–89, 137
PRP injections   188–89
PT. See physical therapist


**R**

radiation   89-90, 92, 118, 123–24,
  183, 219, 225
radiology
  centers   47–48, 121, 208–12
  reports   127, 210–12
  technicians   40, 47–48, 55, 90, 116,
    120–21, 123, 125, 204, 208–9
rectum   53, 75–77, 86–89, 91, 102,
  112–13, 116–17, 130, 132, 135–36,
  142, 170, 173, 199, 211
Reflex Sympathetic Dystrophy.
  See RSD
reproductive organs   89–91, 123–25,
  132, 135, 211, 225

RSD (Reflex Sympathetic Dystrophy)
    81, 83

**S**

sacroiliac joint    106, 109–10
sacrum    19, 30–32, 34–36, 69, 85–87,
    89, 90-1, 93–95, 98, 100–101, 107,
    109–10, 116–17, 126, 129, 138, 149,
    152–53, 197, 207, 240
sciatica    103, 108
skin    65–66, 68, 83, 93, 94, 96–97,
    99–102, 111, 159, 166–67, 183,
    191–92, 197, 207, 209, 216
    breakdown    93–94, 166
    infection    96, 100, 102
SMP (Sympathetically Maintained
    Pain)    36, 81–83, 185
spine    16, 19, 29–30, 31-2, 35-6, 82,
    101, 106–9, 115, 118, 125, 232, 227
standing coccyx x-rays    47–48,
    120–21
steroid injections    79, 133, 163, 183,
    184, 187, 189, 198
stool    20, 53, 75, 77, 87–88, 116–17,
    130, 135, 164, 197
surgeons    86, 102, 137, 196, 198
surgery to remove the tailbone    40,
    49, 70, 74, 79, 85-86, 94-5, 100, 102,
    137, 140–42, 145, 164, 189, 195–200,
    205, 223
Sympathetically Maintained Pain.
    See SMP
sympathetic nerve blocks    38,
    82–83, 184–87, 198
sympathetic nervous system    36,
    79–82, 184–86
    hyperactivity    81–83
symptoms
    tailbone. See tailbone pain
    generalized    88, 91, 95–97
    local    88, 95

**T**

tailbone
    abnormalities    115, 125-27, 134
    abnormal position    18, 38, 41, 60,
        75, 77
    alignment    41–42, 59, 62, 117, 120,
        172
    anatomy    36, 182–83, 198
    arthritis    71-74, 79
    attachments    35–36, 134
    bones    33, 172
    bone spurs    37, 65-7, 70, 117, 172,
        183, 187
    cancer    85-92
    cushions    49, 74, 145, 151–58, 190,
        221, 226, 231
    dislocations    58–64
    excessively-forward    53
    extended    78
    fractures. See fractures
    images    204, 212
    infection    94–95
    injections. See injections
    injuries    38, 53-55, 119, 202, 216,
        218, 225, 237, 239–41
    manipulation    169–73
    MRI images. See MRI
    pain. See tailbone pain
    symptoms    27, 176, 205, 207, 219
    unstable    39–49
    x-rays    24, 39, 47, 117, 225
tailbone pain
    causes    7-137
    treatments    139-200
Tailbone Pain Symptom Checklist
    21
tailboneS, plural term    32, 56
Tarlov cysts    110-11
TB (tuberculosis)    101, 130
tendons    33, 35–36, 61, 102, 112,
    132–33, 142, 170, 188, 196, 217

toilet seat, custom   157
tuberculosis. *See* TB

**U**
urinary bladder   89–91, 96, 99–100,
    112–13, 129, 134, 136, 199, 232
urologist   20, 89, 91, 126, 136–37
uterus   87–89, 112–13, 123, 126, 135,
    199, 210, 213, 232

**V**
variability   32, 55, 62, 75–76

**W**
WBCs (white blood cells)   97–98
weight-bearing   44, 46–47, 56–58,
    64, 66, 68-9, 72–73, 147, 152, 224
white blood cells. *See* WBCs

**X**
x-rays   24, 32–33, 39, 40, 46–49, 51,
    54–55, 63, 65, 68, 72, 75, 87, 89, 97,
    115–121, 130, 182, 187-88, 199,
    207–10, 219, 224–25, 239-40
dynamic. *See* x-rays, seated tailbone
seated tailbone   48–49, 115,
    120–21, 188, 206, 209
sitting-versus-standing   48–49
standard   40, 48, 65, 115–16, 118,
    120

# Free Bonuses for You

For your free copies of any or all of the checklists, handouts, and step-by-step guides mentioned at the end of various chapters of this book, go to: **TailboneDoctor.com/forms**

Below is a list of the free materials that are available for you.

- **Symptoms:** tailbone pain symptom checklist
- **Anatomy:** detailed images and descriptions of tailbone anatomy
- **Unstable joints of the tailbone:** descriptions and details including sitting x-rays
- **Tailbone fractures:** risks and categories
- **Bone spurs:** step-by-step guide to recognizing and diagnosing coccyx bone spurs
- **Cancer:** checklist to screen for cancers of the tailbone region
- **Infections:** checklist to screen for infections of the tailbone region
- **Pain diagram:** where you can document your back, buttock, and tailbone pain
- **Tests:** form where you can document tests you've had done
- **Consults:** form where you can document and track your consults with medical specialists
- **Medications:** List of medications that decrease tailbone pain
- **Injections:** form where you can document which injections you have had and your response to those
- **Coccygectomy:** checklist of tests and treatments for ongoing tailbone pain after coccygectomy
- **Pregnancy/childbirth checklist:** to review with your gynecologist or midwife
- **Children:** template showing typical school Gym Restrictions
- **Insurance:** form to help you track your interactions with your insurance company
- **Legal:** checklist to help you document your tailbone pain in a legal case

# Notes

# Notes

# Notes